25 – 7 – 2010

To Dave

Trust [...] reading [...] of [...] give you a lot of Pleasure

With Best Wishes for now, and the future

Perry Salmon
Author.

One Per Cent

One Per Cent

The Patient Patient

by

Percy Salmon

NOMLAS PRESS

Copyright © Percy Salmon 2005
First published in 2005 by Nomlas Press
147 Pyrles Lane, Loughton
Essex IG10 2NH
www.amolibros.co.uk

Distributed by Gazelle Book Services Limited
Hightown, White Cross Mills, South Rd
Lancaster, England LA1 4XS

The right of Percy Salmon to be identified as the author of the work has been asserted herein in accordance with the Copyright, Designs and Patents Act 1988.

All rights reserved. This book is sold subject to the condition that it shall not, by way of trade or otherwise, be lent, resold, hired out or otherwise circulated without the publisher's prior consent in any form of binding or cover other than that in which it is published and without a similar condition including this condition being imposed on the subsequent purchaser.

British Library Cataloguing in Publication Data
A catalogue record for this book is available from the British Library

ISBN 0-9540055-1-1

Typeset by Amolibros, Milverton, Somerset
This book production has been managed by Amolibros
Printed and bound by Advance Book Printing, Oxford, England

Introduction

First and foremost, I must make it quite clear that any criticism, fault-finding, description of conditions or suggested improvements, which the reader will find as the pages of *One Per Cent* are turned, are never in any way to be read as being suggestive of unsatisfactory treatment or an undisciplined approach to my well-being and care.

I am most sincere when I state categorically that having been in several different hospitals, as both patient and visitor, I have found that quick remedial treatments are never the norm, with patience and unpredictability being the operative words.

I doubt that I was a model patient; if I were I would imagine everything would have gone like clockwork. I can assure you that as you follow my daily diary in and out of Holly House Hospital, you will find my problem proved to be far from straightforward.

The usual procedure for a knee replacement has improved beyond all recognition over recent years, with operations and care so advanced that when you are told "between *fourteen* and *sixteen days*"—you assume that your clearance to go home is on the cards within that time frame. Normal post-operative care and attention, if there are no complications, should move smoothly along as follows:-

1   Intravenous infusion for the first twenty-four to forty-eight hours.

2. Three doses of intravenous antibiotics (usually cefuroxine 750 mgs) are administered.
3. CLEXANE. (The injection to protect against DVT) 20-40 i.u. subcutaneous daily until discharge. This can be given in any area of the body—including the stomach. It is given with a small needle just under the skin, then ASPIRIN, 75 mgs daily until the first Outpatient appointment (usually four to six weeks after discharge).
4. A blood transfusion of 2 – 4 units can be administered either pre- or post-operatively. A blood test for haemoglobin (HB) will be checked forty-eight hours post-operatively and a further transfusion administered if the HB is below 9 gms.
5. Sutures or clips are removed fourteen days post-operatively.
6. Physiotherapy starts the day after the operation; this includes the CPM exercises, walking, depending on the patient's improvement—the staircase.

I want to dedicate this book to all the staff who have had anything to do with my various operations. This includes anyone who has played a part in keeping me in such good spirits on my long road to recovery.

Certainly I know this covers many professionals attached to Holly House Hospital and its daily routine of endless comings and goings.

There are many unsung heroes and heroines; I like to think that without their help perhaps I might not be in a position to say this small thank you to them.

Holly House Hospital has been established for over twenty-four years, and is known locally for its friendly welcome and high standards of nursing care. Readers wanting to know more about Holly House can visit their website: www.hollyhouse-hospital.co.uk.

A Patient Beginning

An appointment on Saturday, 26th May 2001 with Mr McAuliffe, one of the orthopaedic surgeons at Holly House Hospital was not going to be as straightforward as I had first imagined. I knew my left knee had been playing me up for some time and at the back of my mind was the thought that it might mean more attention than I had at first considered. It was now nearly ten years since I had had an arthroscopy operation and over the subsequent years the leg had suffered plenty of abuse—especially when you think that this leg of mine had been the front and landing one when I had bowled for something like twenty-five summers playing cricket for the village team. After four x-rays had been taken I was seated in front of Mr McAuliffe who proceeded to show and tell me that the knee was in a right mess—the only way forward would be to have a total knee replacement. He immediately got out his diary to find suitable dates for us both.

I told him straightaway that I expected to have a pretty busy summer and would much prefer a date perhaps towards the end of it, reminding him also that I wanted to go to New Zealand in the early part of 2002 to watch the England cricket team with other supporters, leaving in mid-February. Mr McAuliffe said nothing, just nodding in response to my remarks. So the 6th September was fixed for my operation.

I had to arrange with my insurance company that it was all right for this to go ahead, and to be confirmed within a few days by Credit Control in the Accounts Department of the hospital. I had every reason to expect an excellent replacement being accomplished for this would be the third stainless steel joint he had fitted. I had had a left-hip replacement done in 1995 and my right knee in 1998 and through subsequent years they really had been a splendid advert for the treatment of replacement joints. Whatever you do you don't treat them as though they must be handled with care but trust them.

September 5th

An appointment with the various departments to make sure all my working parts were in good nick. These and the ECG machine were to make sure that whilst I was under anaesthetic, during the operation the next day, nothing would be left to chance. All these check-ups began at 11.30 a.m. and were finished by 13.50 in the afternoon.

Accounts had also finally cleared me for the go-ahead and later I received a telephone call from one of the Admission Nurses that all my tests were fine. The operation goes ahead tomorrow.

September 6th

I had been looking after my neighbour's dog Bruce, so one of the first jobs this morning was to take him for his last walk with me—then wait for the new temporary charges to come and collect him.

A taxi up to Holly House Hospital where I booked into Reception and was taken to Room 157 and made to feel at ease by the admission staff. Time now 11.30 a.m.

Mr McAuliffe came to see me in the early afternoon, gave me some more assurances, signed on the dotted line and marked my left leg with a black pen, confirming that I would be going down to theatre later on in the afternoon.

Another very important person associated with the operation also paid me a visit, Mr Dodd the anaesthetist, whom I knew already from my previous visits; he was ready for me when the porter and nurse delivered me to his waiting area at 17.45.

As I lay on the bed prior to his sending me to sleep, the pre-op room had an artist's drawing above my head of a country scene of farmyard animals, farm workers and farm paraphernalia. (Little did I know then that I was to come almost to know this picture off by heart!)

Back in Room 157 approximately just before 21.00 with priority attention given to me at this stage since I had just had major surgery—as I was assured this indeed was. I have had a fair bit of pain in the night—and it is only certain times during this time that painkillers are allowed, so you have to grin and bear it. Then of course when you are rewarded it does not work as quickly as rubbing your hands together. I had to wait but, fortunately, as I could now take fluids, I was allowed a cuppa and a piece of toast.

September 7th

8.15 a.m.—one of the first jobs of the day staff is to change the dressings that already had been changed by the night staff together with another change of sheets as these have been soiled again with blood. What was also going to be the norm for the rest of my stay was having my observations done at intervals during the day: blood pressure, temperature, pulse, injections— just some of the vital chores concerning a patient's well-being.

Breakfast—cereals, toast and marmalade. Next a wash, shave and brush-up. Order for a daily newspaper and delivered straight to your bed.

Later in the morning I was taken down to the Radiology Department for a couple of x-rays; these were quickly developed and handed to the nurse who came along with us—then back to 157—these placed in my chart-holder attached to the bottom part of the bed rail.

Early afternoon, Mr McAuliffe called in to tell me that everything had gone according to plan—also took a quick glance at the x-ray plates—then told me it is important that I use the machine to get the knee moving again as quickly as possible.

I had already met the Mrs Moppses who all seemed to be a jolly bunch and, as I found as time passed, no task was either too large or small for their capabilities, their positive attitude designed to get patients up and about again as quick as shaking their mops out. Another person who had made my acquaintance during the morning was the physiotherapist who came in at 15.00 with the CPM—compulsive passive movement machine. I'll try to describe it. It is like a giant foot pump where your whole leg is lifted on, laid out straight, then strapped to it with Velcro straps leaving an area where your knee joint can move freely with the movement of the CPM. There is also a stop and start button which regulates the degrees; it can go to well over 100 degrees which is well beyond the 90 degrees the physio has in mind for you. Agreeing that 25 degrees would be a good starter and a half hour would be fine, I made a start.

Just below the top layer of metal stitches in the lower part of my thigh, a drain pipe had been inserted to take away the wastage (as I would call it) which the body tends to sort out following the intake of fluids not only by mouth but also through the drip feed perched up on the wheelie seven-foot frame, allowing your blood to return to a good clean healthy circulation—for as I was to find out, blood tests were imperative in making sure the old ticker received only the best quality passing through. The drainpipe, by the way, passing into a jam jar, was attached to the frame of the bed.

Through the day I was fussed over as if I had been royalty and this was only my first full day of meals. I had a choice of several splendid menus and the waitresses who came with them always brought their cheerful smiles with them, often accompanied by a remark which you had to be on the same wavelength to appreciate—this without a doubt good healthy 'get better' medicine. Just after lights out I asked if I could have a sleeping tablet to send me to sleep. It worked like magic.

September 8th

I had to have a change of sheets in the night as the drainpipe had come out and had made a right mess. No doubt on instructions from Mr McAuliffe, the resident doctor has told me that we can now leave it out altogether and, as there had been hardly any inflow into the jar, this was good thinking. I was happy, for now I could turn about in the bed.

During the day there had been lots of traffic moving up and down the corridor and also into and out of rooms here on Cedar Ward, especially lots of day patients who came in, had their ops, settled down, recovered and then went home.

I had to have the dressing changed four or five times as this one particular place kept oozing blood. It seemed to be about four stitches down where they had not quite been placed equal distances apart.

Mr McAuliffe had been in to see me and agreed with the staff that I was to keep off the CPM—yes I could do some walking—together with some exercises on the bed. This being Saturday, new staff had taken over the Monday-to-Friday duties of cleaning ladies, waitresses, etc. There was also a different physiotherapist, and when she saw me for the first time I straightaway referred to her as a sergeant major, which I might add did not upset her at all. In fact she was most upset because she could not do much for me except take me for a walk along the corridor.

I asked if I could have a sleeping tablet later, which knocked me out just before 23.00.

September 9th

Breakfast—I am now having a couple of poached eggs on two pieces of toast with a couple of slices extra with marmalade.

The physiotherapist arrived and immediately said, 'It's best to leave the machine today,' so I did some walking with a frame. Mr McAuliffe called in during the afternoon and said he wants me to get back on the CPM, saying, 'Put him back on the machine, for the blood is better out than in,' making sure that the staff and two nurses present heard what he said. 'Get it bending,' he concluded. When I came off the machine just before our dinner was brought in, the blood had started weeping through again. The CPM—I am now up to fifty-two degrees.

I had had my meal and tablets and was doing some writing when I first heard the noise coming from the wall at the bottom of the bed. I must have dozed off then and was awakened by the waitress bringing in my late night drink—a cup of hot chocolate.

As I had the telly on, other noises were banished from my now very drowsy grey cells. It was not until I turned the telly off at 21.55 that the noise I had heard earlier came back to remind me that all was not well with my neighbour in the next room. I rang the buzzer, which had an immediate response from not only the two night nurses on duty but also the sister who wanted to know what was up. I said, 'I'm pretty sure there's something amiss in the room next door—if you listen you will hear it the same as me.' All with one voice they said, 'Yes, there is something,' and again in unison, 'But the next room is empty—Mrs So and So went home earlier in the afternoon.'

It was then that I noticed a very slight movement against the wall in question. I then knew that I had solved the enigma, saying to the three night staff, 'Take a close look at the wall just up from the carpet on the floor.' The sister twigged it straightaway, going straight to the nearest plug point and turning off the CPM machine—for indeed this is exactly what was causing the noise. When it had been removed after my exercises it had been placed horizontally against the wall but in an upright position so its movements were travelling backwards and forwards along the wallpaper. Both machine and wallpaper were almost an identical colour and with the CPM movement so very slow this made it difficult to observe. I then relaxed altogether and had a restful night, with the mystery of my intruder well and truly solved.

September 10th

About an hour after breakfast when a little peace had settled in the various rooms, the physiotherapist had called to say that orders confirmed I was to get back on the CPM regardless of the little loss of blood. It was not long before the sheets were receiving a fair amount of blood, so all the sheets, including dressings were changed—it appears that I now had low blood pressure. I was doing quite well on the CPM for I was now up to sixty-seven degrees and feeling quite comfortable. It was just the place where the metal stitches were that seemed to be stopping progress.

After lunch Mr McAuliffe called in with the day sister and gave some new instructions saying, 'Keep the CPM going and also the walking.' The physiotherapist put me back on the machine after I had gone for a walk and now that I was walking with the arm crutches, I was quite confident I was up with the schedule.

September 11th

I had had a decent night with only just a tiny weeping of blood, but still everything was changed, the dressings, the lot. Already you could see where the lower stitches were healing nicely.

This was about the only time I had my breakfast sent up wrongly. This was quickly sorted out by the chef in charge that particular day.

I had found that my occupation of writing letters was going to help me through my hospital stay and had just started a letter to a couple I knew in Cornwall. The time—just before 9.00 a.m. One of the nurses rushed in and said, 'Haven't you got the telly on, Perc?' She went immediately to the set and turned it on, continuing, 'A plane has crashed into the World Trade Centre in New York.' We then both looked in amazement as the cameras picked up another aircraft and we watched it crash into another skyscraper. I must confess I don't expect to see anything like this again in my lifetime; within an hour, a third plane had crashed into the Pentagon. This was all the devilish work of terrorists.

Had a gentle day with the physiotherapist. I have been for a couple of walks and on the CPM for nearly two hours. The afternoon session completed just before 18.00 when I had reached seventy degrees.

I was now suffering with my blood, which seemed to be playing up most staff including the sisters—there appeared to be an iron deficiency. However, I was pleased with the day's progress—yet at the back of my mind was so much sympathy for all those thousands who had lost their lives in New York; it was a talking point when the waitresses and night staff arrived for their duties.

A sleeping tablet just before lights out sent me—I am sure—into a good night's rest.

September 12th

As the terrorist attack was again the talking point first thing, I had to keep up with the latest news—to keep not only the staff informed but myself—by turning on the television, even the night sister with the trolley at 6.15am—of the 911 murders as it was to become known. It seemed one particular group of Arabs seemed to be the instigators with the leader known as Bin Laden. The approximate number of people dead at this time was given as over 5,000. Through the rest of the day I knew the three suicide planes and their routes to destruction off by heart.

I had had my breakfast and was wondering what the pains were around my tummy with lots of unfamiliar noises going on. The physiotherapist arrived and as soon as I started moving about so I started bringing up the wind. I walked and did some staircase exercises with her and thought I now had her sympathy—not so!! Straight onto the CPM, which made me even more uncomfortable. Finally, I rang the staff nurse, telling her my indigestion was getting out of hand and could she get me some bicarbonate of soda, as this always does the trick for me when I get wind at home. However, a hot peppermint drink arrived which helped the situation but only temporarily and the pain continued with me for the rest of the day. By the end of the CPM session I had now reached seventy-seven degrees and had held it for some ten minutes.

Even though the night sister decided to change my iron

tablets and give me a couple of sleeping tablets to send me off—I still had a shocking night.

September 13th

I had not improved at all and after I ate my breakfast, washed, shaved, etc. I thought that as a new physio had started, I would be relieved of some of the regular duties. Not so, walking and CPM, but the belching continued wherever I was exercising. One of the senior staff seemed to think the reason for the indigestion could well be that the iron tablet I was taking did not work with the Voltarol tablet I was taking for my arthritis problems.

By the time dinner arrived later in the day, not only had I moved the CPM up to and held seventy-seven degrees but had moved up to eighty-two degrees. This had not stopped the occasional leaking of blood which meant I had to have the dressing changed. Thursday is usually a busy day for operations and it was not until 21.15 that Mr McAuliffe called in to see how I was getting on. He picked up my notes which told him or rather confirmed what he had been told, that my indigestion had not improved. He said, 'I think what we should do is stop the Voltarol.' Taking a quick look at the wound after removing part of the dressing, he continued, 'It's still weeping then?'

September 14th

Not a very good night for I had the deuce of a job to get to sleep owing to the rumblings in my tummy. The night staff changed my dressing; after I had carried out my regular ablutions and was doing some bed exercises one of the nurses came in and looked at me, evidently reported something to the staff nurse in charge, and the next thing I had the Resident

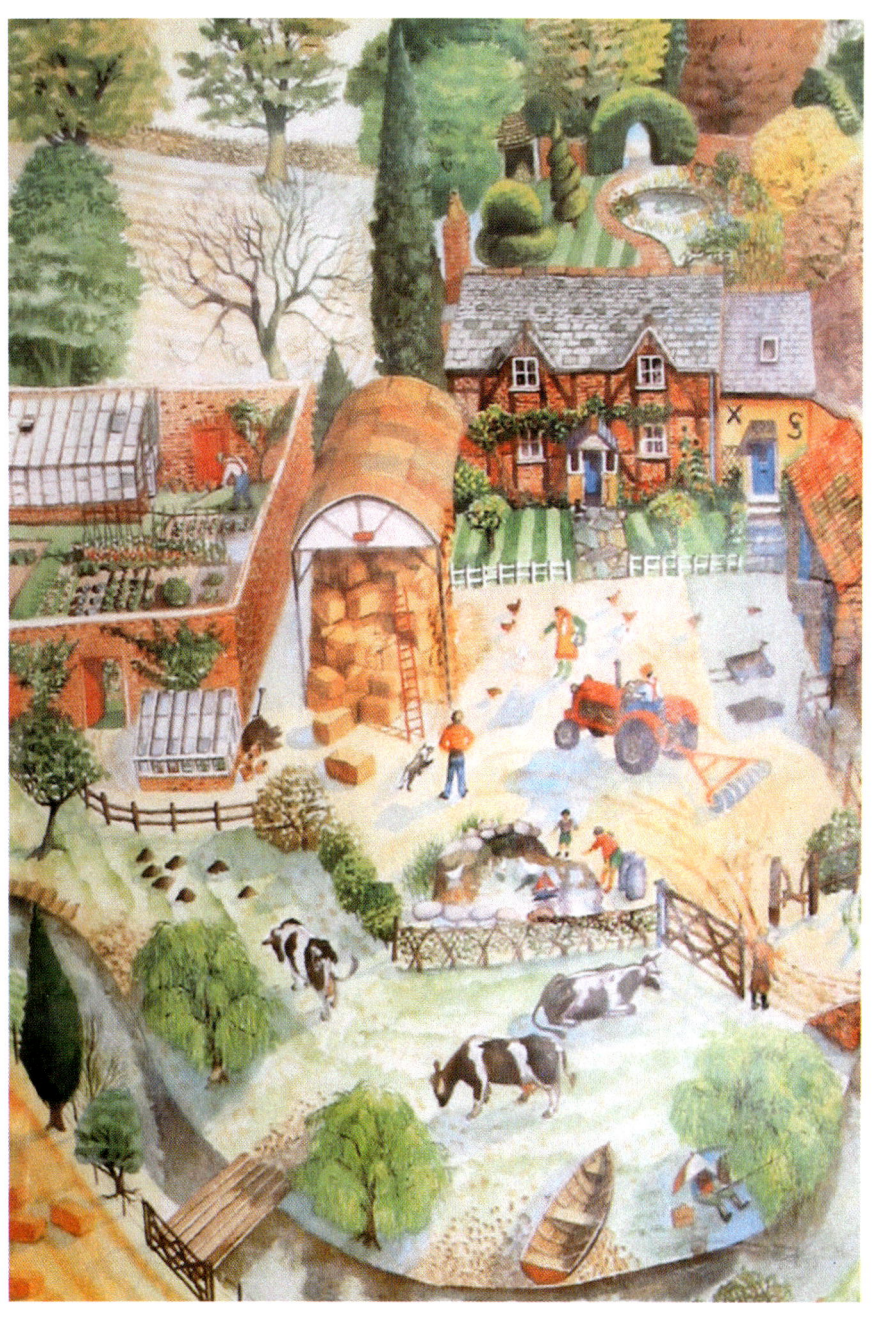

Holly House Hospital had this ceiling in their Recovery Room. Reproduced here by kind permission of Robin Wilcox.

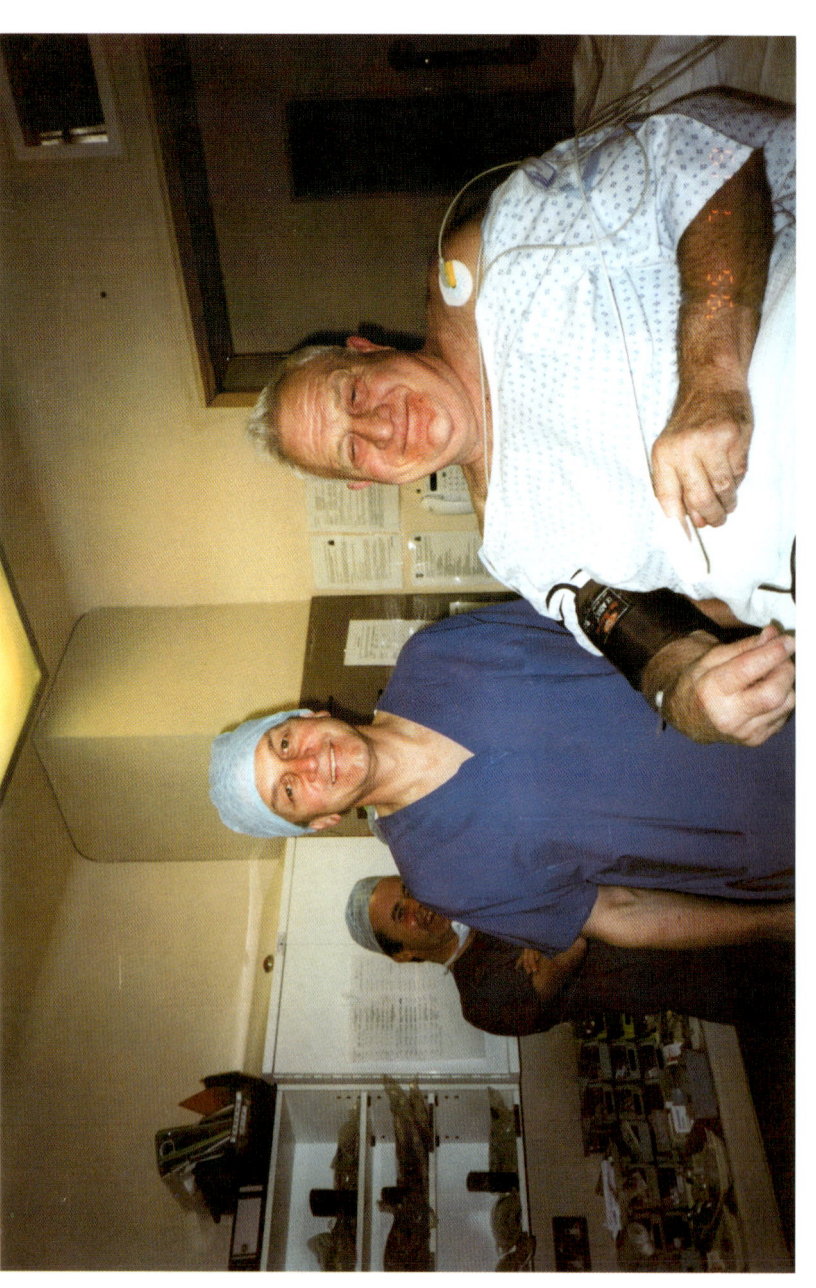

Mr McAuliffe and Mr Dodds get ready to do Percy's op.

Doctor in the room with the ECG machine, approximately 10.30 a.m.

The physio arrived: a walk to the staircase, up and down a few times then back on the CPM. The luncheon arrives near enough to 12.00 and at just about this time a hot milky drink turned up for my indigestion and on the plate for my dessert was an ice cream—'not a successful combination'.

I am now comfortable walking by myself, for not only is it helping my leg get stronger but also getting rid of the wind. As I pass each room which has an inmate in, I apologise for being so inconsiderate and saying that I shall be glad when it's sorted out. One person who also shall be nameless said, 'And so shall we.'

I continued however with my correspondence. Not only letters, but also some proof-reading. At 17.30 I came off the CPM for the last time today having reached eighty-five degrees and feeling comfortable, having been attached to it since 16.30.

Just before 20.00 Mr McAuliffe called in and asked how I was. I was quite honest with him when I said a good friend of mine, a retired senior staff nurse, had heard all about my symptoms and said I should be treated with something for lower down in the stomach. I am never sure how he feels about me interfering—but as was usual all I received was a grin that quickly appeared and just as quickly disappeared, and, 'Let's see what it's like tomorrow.'

Lights out and a couple of sleeping tablets soon sent me off.

September 15th

The weekend staff have arrived and 7.30 the early morning cuppa trolley is soon on the way. Some do not participate but I started with it from day one and now I look forward to it together with a couple of Rich Tea biscuits. The breakfast I had ordered from the night before duly came at 8.15 a.m.—cereals and toast—but I hardly touched anything. The indigestion is still around and I'm sure if it is affecting the blood pressure problem I am suffering from. Surely it's time now after several days—I should be showing an improvement.

The physio arrived at 9.40 and without doing any walking exercises I went straight on the CPM and stayed on it until after 11.00—now up to eighty-seven degrees and holding it for a few minutes. As one of the staff nurses is not quite so busy I ask her if I can see the RD about my wind; he duly arrives. I told him about the Voltarol—he goes and gets his own chart saying I should have to keep on the iron tablets until blood is back to normal—then I can restart the Voltarol—it is now 0.9; whatever that might mean but it should be much lower than that. He also mentioned I looked pale, and did I get out of breath quickly? Among the questions asked was—did I suffer with wind normally?—how long had I had blood problems?

Just after my lunch, which I only made a token gesture at eating, Mr McAuliffe arrives, 'How do you feel?' I replied, 'You must know how I feel if I am not eating anything. Do you think you ought to change the iron tablets I am taking?' At the back of my mind was the tablet which Sue had mentioned beginning with L but for the life of me I could not remember its full name. (Sue is a retired nursing officer from Whipps Cross Hospital.)

Between 16.00 and 17.20, I very gently eased my way up to eighty degrees on the CPM. Quite a few visitors had come to see me, including a good friend of mine who lives round the corner on the Knighton Estate, who I found to be a jolly good visitor. Unfortunately he had problems of his own for he was suffering from Parkinson's Disease—which at times made me feel really sorry for him, especially when he stood up and was unable to get his legs working with his brain. Still, he always looked forward to popping in to see me regardless of the weather or his health.

What I also know is that my knee is mighty painful.

September 16th

I have marked up a better night—with my indigestion improved.

7.20 a.m. the early morning cuppa arrives with most of the weekend staff already moving about. In fact one of the sisters who went past I really did not recognise because she was dressed up for something special. There had been a troublesome night with a patient in a nearby room—am not clear if this was connected, but if so the sight of our sister looking like this would cheer up the most unhappy room occupant.

By 8.30 a.m. I had received and eaten my breakfast. Is my appetite coming back for I had eaten and enjoyed two poached eggs on toast? All the morning tasks had been accomplished too including my back having some special attention with some talc—which I cannot stand; however, the nurse did this for a bit of devilment because she knows that aftershaves, etc, are vetoed by me.

The physiotherapist arrived and after reading my notes and following instructions that the knee was swollen and running hot, not only was I to go on the CPM but also have an ice pack attached to the knee in question. 'Won't it interfere with the movement of the CPM?' 'No, not at all if the ice pack is put on correctly.' So a nurse was detailed to change the water every twenty minutes, so for an hour and twenty minutes I had to keep an eye open—not only watching the dials on the machine but also the ice pack. The CPM up to eighty-eight degrees and holding, and my weather eye on the clock—

everything came off, including another new dressing which had only been changed earlier when the sheets had been changed.

At 12.10 my lunch arrived and I'm pleased to say I ate the lot. No, I was not overdoing things for I knew that if I over-indulged with all the delicious menus that I could select from, this would be of no benefit to me at all, so I chose good healthy foods including what I had just enjoyed—a salad and fruit dessert.

Straightaway I decided to have a walk along the corridor and noticed that there were not too many patients in, in fact just eight rooms were occupied.

15.00 I was back on the CPM and the ice pack, with an agency nurse who was looking after me. She would not admit it but you could see that this was probably the first one she had ever seen—a machine strange to me too. Between us we made a fair job of this and with the eighty-eight degrees I held for some twenty minutes I was well pleased with the afternoon. Mind you, I had to have another dressing put on as the discharge had started again. It was in the same place each time and did not look like it was healing up. As I lay there thinking of all sorts of ways to try to seal this small aperture, one method I had considered was asking Mr McAuliffe why I couldn't have a piece of skin grafted over and I knew a place around my buttocks which was available where this would not be missed!

19.40—a lot of blood had started oozing through the dressing and as about this time there are changeovers going on regards duties, staff coming on and going off. It is awkward ones like myself who always seem to want attention with dressing changes. So until there was more peace and quiet I asked for some Micropore, which I came to find was magical stuff and adhered to the skin but never harmed it—peeling off as quickly as it was put on. Two different sorts were available, and I was to find that keeping a particular type in my locker was useful as it was always ready then for the nurses who came in. In fact as my stay continued so nurses would pop in and take some ready Elastoplast from my stores saying, 'I'll bring anther roll in when I'm passing.' I might also say at this stage that I also collected the little plastic pots for pills and tablets which did not take up too much space for they fitted into one another like a concertina. These came from the trolley which I am sure was the same one that was around when I paid my very first visit back at the end of 1992. It had an unmistakable note of its own as it was trundled backwards and forwards along the corridors carrying patients' medicines to help speed their recovery.

Lights out and one of the busy-bee night nurses had arrived and as there were not too many patients, these were the occasions when the nurses proved their worth, because not only are they equipped to care for patients, sick or otherwise, but also to listen to personal tales of and sensitive stuff. Being sympathetic—not necessarily advising but just comforting a patient—not only makes that person feel important but gives him a stronger will to get better as it releases stored-up feelings. So a good nurse is not only a strong-willed one—with her own problems stored away; she provides help to stimulate others in need—more often than not mentioning some other patient in the room a few doors down who is much worse off. 'My, this is really get-up-and-go medicine.' I overheard this same nurse having an electrifying chat to a patient the next day and what a change in that patient!

Yes, every nurse has this valuable attribute and I am sure as they get more senior this seems to be a paramount part of their qualifications for being a better nurse.

Lights out. I asked if I could have a couple of sleeping tablets as well as a couple of painkillers as I am getting quite a few pains around the repaired knee.

September 17th

It is now eleven days since my operation. It seemed that the majority are on their way after this type of knee replacement within fourteen days—but, goodness knows, I would have to make some vast improvement in the next couple of days, with a magician doing more than wave his wand to get me out, healed and walking. I had a pretty good night with all my tablets doing their job—the trolley on the move at 6.15 a.m.

I had my early morning cuppa, breakfast, wash, shave and had started reading the morning paper after a quick walk along the corridor—time approximately 9.30 a.m. when the physio arrived. I told her I had had a walk and my wind had all flared up again—and I told her no way did I want to go on the CPM for, as I have marked up in the diary, I was belching like a trooper. I really thought that it had settled down but whatever it was, a pocket of wind had been laying dormant somewhere, I reckoned.

It was not long after this that Mr McAuliffe arrived to tell me that a doctor specialist for gastric problems would be coming along to see me. The sister on duty said I must continue with the CPM machine and try to improve on what I had done so far with the degrees of bending I was achieving, also endorsed by the physiotherapist. So back I went and at 11.35 a.m. while reading the newspaper, doing the crossword, I cracked it—ninety degrees, and holding it for some ten minutes.

Just before our lunch break a visit from the RD who took some blood, putting it in a phial with labelling saying, 'We will get this done straightaway.'—Not so!

After lunch at 12.40, another doctor called a Gastroenterologist arrived to say I have to pop on the urology machine to find out where all the gas is coming from—that's tomorrow. Later in the afternoon I had a walk up and down the corridor a few times; as I had hardly eaten anything, it was reasonably peaceful as I walked along minding my own business—but still enquiring after people's health in some of the rooms I was passing. Some I introduced myself to which got an immediate response, telling me their first names in an instant and straightaway asking about my health and was everything going all right as I was walking about? Then would follow their health, how long since the op, where they came from and quite a few times they knew someone I knew or vice versa, around the district. Just before dinner a visit from the sister to tell me about my blood count—it is 10.4—that is good. A change of dressing at 21.45 started the blood off again and all the sheets had to be changed once more.

September 18th

I had a rough night although I had taken two painkillers and also sleeping tablets. Cuppa arrived at 7.20. But, as I have to go on the ultrasound machine early afternoon—no breakfast. I had taken another tablet for indigestion: Losec—it sounds as if this is the tablet I have heard mentioned by my retired friend and staff nurse Sue.

The doctor called to see me at 13.45 and I'm back in Room 157 at 14.30 having had a jelly-like substance spread around my stomach area. A Dr Greaves I believe who attended me. My poor old leg is certainly suffering though for it's like a furnace—it's bending all right as I sit on the edge of the bed, but when I lay flat on the bed it's not so good. Had a visit from my friend who stayed until just before dinner. This I really enjoyed for it seemed as though the aches and pains I had been having were disappearing. I did some walking not only along the corridor but also quite a few times up and down the staircase, which did not do the knee much good later—

for when the night sister came round with the trolley she did not like the look of my knee and straightaway fetched the RD in to see me. He did not even feel it—just looked at it, saying, 'It needs more exercising.'

September 19th

The night staff are on the move at 6.00 a.m. One of the nurses on duty tells me she lives just around the corner from me in Pyrles Lane. Early morning cuppa arrives together with the breakfast at 8.00 a.m. I ate everything including the extra baked beans I had received on my plate. It's a dreadful day outside for it's pouring with rain.

As there appears to be a shortage of physios, I asked one of the nurses to put me on the CPM, for if as the RD suggested, it was exercise that was required then I'd better be getting on with it—there was no more willing patient than myself to co-operate with this way of thinking. The dressing had been changed earlier but was still oozing as I went on gradually to ninety-five degrees and held it there for some time. I enjoyed my lunch. Early afternoon I went for a walk for some twenty minutes, then a staff nurse put me on the CPM where I started in the high eighties and finished on ninety-five degrees.

I was glad when the nurse came and took it away, for the knee ached like hell. It was after late night drinks that Mr McAuliffe called round to tell me that he is not happy with the blood that keeps oozing from the wound saying, 'I think you had better keep off the machine for a couple of days and this might help to stop the flow of blood.' He also told me, as most sports people know, he is the Medical Officer for West Ham FC, that he had given the once-over to a well-known defender who might be joining a rival team, Spurs, from

Southampton. Of course I did not even ask what might the applicant be suffering from or his name, but you may depend on it, even if I had asked, sure thing, I would have had a negative response. He continued telling me, 'It's most important that the area where the blood is coming from heals up—then we can take the stitches out.' Asking the sister how long was it now since the operation? Her response: 'It's now thirteen days,' after looking at my chart. I am pretty sure that two sleeping tablets and two painkillers later I was soon asleep.

September 20th

I had a rough night as through the night I asked the night sister for a couple more painkillers. The pain seems to be down in the knee. She also made me a cuppa and chatted whilst I went off to sleep.

After morning observations, the sheets had to be changed again for more blood had come through the new dressing that I'd had put on. 10.30, mid-morning, a swab had been taken to see if I was growing anything. This little phial went straight down to the Pathology Department, the results to be known in the morning.

The physio had been informed of the situation but I could go for a walk, also bed-stretching exercises every hour on the bed and bedside were allowed.

Luncheon: I had had the lot today—ham, eggs, chips, etc. and fruit dessert. More exercises at 15.30—went for a walk. One of the patients I was chatting to was Peter who, it appeared, had been to several places I had visited in recent years around part of the globe. After dinner—more walking and found that after a busy day of exercising at 21.00 I had to have a change of dressing for it was in a bloody mess. Later, sleeping tablets and painkillers.

September 21st

After a pretty good night the message has come through that the dressing is to stay on. 7.00 a.m. the nurse has just completed the observations. Early morning cuppa arrives at 7.30 a.m. 8.15 a.m.—breakfast—when I ate everything including a spare piece of toast. Staff nurse informs me that the dressing has still to stay on. The physiotherapist arrives and after doing some leg exercises on the bed, has opened up the wound and has now started the blood oozing again—the staff nurse who'd earlier said not to was soon on the scene changing the dressing.

Lunch break and being as it was Friday I had decided to have a piece of haddock with chips—very nice, followed by a fruit dessert.

I must say I had a very nice surprise with a visitor who came in to see me—our flower lady whom I associate with the church at High Beech who tells me that she works here in the Holly House Hospital Path Lab and seeing my name on the specimen sent in for examination put two and two together and guessed correctly that it was me.

Had several walks and chats with various room occupants, including an exercise with another patient on the staircase—both of us I might add reasonably accomplished now—especially myself now completing my sixteenth day. Still taking my sleeping tablets which I find are a godsend in sending me off—mind you, though, I cannot recall having been disturbed by any patients with any sleeping disorders.

September 22nd

I have had a bad night as I have had a pain down one side of my leg for most of the night—that's when I was awake. As there was the possibility of me going home today as scheduled there is not much likelihood of that, with niggling pains like this causing problems, no doubt. Day sister came in to say that the result of the swab taken on Thursday should be with us this morning. In fact, this same sister gave my back a real good lathering and towelling whilst chatting to me. She also told me that Mr McAuliffe is coming to see me either before his consultant's appointments or after operations this afternoon. About mid-morning the same sister came along and took all the stitches out—must have been well over forty. Where the healing had gone according to plan, the area looked quite pleasant to look at, but where the blood was oozing from seemed rough and puffy. Sister seemed pleased and said, 'You know, Percy, for all the harsh treatment it's had, it's coming along fine. The swab has also come back—and, yes, Mr Mac knows about this and has put you on two antibiotics to be taken straightaway—then two later on.'

After lunch, he arrived at approximately 12.45, telling me that there is nothing to worry about, for it will soon clear up with the tablets prescribed. No exercise on the staircase, just do some gentle exercises on the bed and walking along the corridor. Second lot of antibiotics at 22.00. By this, my sixteenth day, I had got to know a lot of the waitresses by their first names and what a super bunch they were, great for leg-pulling, in a cheerful kind, considerate, gentle, explosive way—a you-don't-want-to-go-home attitude from most of them. I must include all the other staff as well, whilst I am concentrating on the fact that the way to a man's heart is via his tummy.

September 23rd

Rotten night again, from 5.00 a.m. I could not get back to sleep. Early morning cuppa at 7.20. When breakfast arrived, I ate most everything that the waitresses had brought in. By

8.40 a.m. I had completed all my ablutions when one of the staff nurses came along and said, 'How about giving your feet a good soak?' As there were three patients going home this morning, I said, 'Could I say ta-ta to them first?' wondering what had I done to deserve this treatment. Sure thing when I got back to Room 157, I was followed in with a bowl of hot water, the staff nurse saying, 'We'll leave them to soak for a while and then I'll be back.' It was quite some time before the nurse remembered that she had left a patient soaking his feet; they had now emerged while I attempted to dry them myself: a scurry of feet, the towel was whipped out—a splendid job was done in drying them—and then another remark that surprised me: 'We'll leave them out to air.' It was not long before I had my slippers back on, also my clean stockings, via another nurse; especially important as the physiotherapist had arrived and wanted to do some walking exercises with me along the corridor. Whilst doing this, we bumped into not only Mr Mac but also Mr Philps, another surgeon who was working here with private patients, those with prostate concerns. He'd looked after me at Whipps Cross Hospital, so we knew one another. Asking me what I was doing here, I told him: 'I expect Mr McAuliffe to get me going on two good knees to see the test matches in New Zealand.' 'Good luck,' he said, this chap also a very busy consultant surgeon.

12.00 I enjoyed my lunch: roast pork, calabrese, boiled potatoes and roasted ones with apple jelly, then the dessert was apple crunch with a fair helping of custard. The physiotherapist had confirmed what I was feeling—an improvement was on the way—and I was enjoying the buzz around me, especially when later in the afternoon, on the telly, West Ham was to beat Newcastle 3–0. It was after my evening meal that the sister on duty popped in to see me, asking me that as I had had two knees replaced, would I like to pop into

Room 143 and have a chat with the patient named Eric there, who was having them done both at once. 'I'll think about it if that's all right.' I dare say the reason why the sister had asked me was because I had now made a bit of a reputation for myself by popping into various patients' rooms and cheering them up with a few of the stories I had gathered over the years. I'm happy to say that everyone enjoyed my visits—well I like to think they had approved of my company. Dwelling over this for some time, I decided that I would pay him a call, so knocked on his door, to find him expecting me, saying, 'You must be Percy.' He was a chap about my age and I asked him straightaway, 'Why did you want to have them both done at the same time?'

He replied, 'Well, the wife and I worked it out that, if I went ahead and had them both done, as they both needed replacing, it was going to be much cheaper cost-wise than having them done separately.'

It was at this point that I said to him, 'I am sure the sister told you that I had something like four years in between replacements, so could not say how you are going to cope with having them both done at the same time. However what I did find was that, when I was either sitting on the bed or table or something similar, I would always swing them both together, and found that while I was exercising one the other was being exercised automatically, even sitting on the bed—though difficult. I tended to do any movement in unison with the other leg, if that's any help.'

Whatever I said, he seemed to approve of what I had to say, so I went on to ask him how he had come to get his knees in disrepair like this—building trade, heavy manual duties or the like? 'No, throughout my life I have been much involved with Cossack dancing.'

'Whew, wow!!' Wishing him the best of luck, I went back

to my room, thinking what an interesting job Mr Mac has and wondering what goes through his mind when he has people in for their pre-op interviews. Late-night drinks arrived. Staff nurse arrived with pills at about 23.00.

September 24th

Most of the general duties all completed by 9.00 a.m. With everything seemingly under control I was out walking when the physio arrived to tell me that Mr Mac had phoned to say that walking up and down the staircase is not to be one of the exercises for the time being. 12.00—I was now beginning to revert to what I was used to having at home—cream crackers with cheese, but here one received as many as four different cheeses together with tasty pieces of celery and frequently dressed round with an assortment of lettuce leaves. Mr Mac arrives with the sister on duty to say, after looking at the wound, 'You can go home the day after tomorrow.' That will be Wednesday, I thought. Shortly after this there was a bit of a kafuffle for sister came in to ask if she left some keys in here—for they were the ones to the drug store along the corridor. One of the nurses also came in asking about them. They were very important things to lose and you could understand the sister's concern. I suggested to her that, as Mr Mac had been in this room at the same time, perhaps he had picked them up—this suggestion was relayed back to him and it appeared that he had them in his pockets. No, I can't tell you if this was really true but this is how it came back to me. The rest of the day went along smoothly. I found that by leaving the door slightly open you can hear the movements of other rooms' occupants and am quite sure that Eric had gone down for his operation about 13.00 and came back about 17.30. As I have mentioned before that is no time for paying visits to another patient—and I am always very surprised that relatives are unable to understand this when it comes to their loved ones—but made a note that I would pop in to see him tomorrow and see how he was progressing following his major surgery.

I was now taking my last two antibiotics still at 22.00 and also the sleeping tablets which I was most grateful for. Tomorrow, I must inform various people about coming home on Wednesday. I was still having the dressing done for me so I knew that this would be a task that I had to master for myself—but fortunately I knew I could take care of this obligation and could not see any reason why I needed help as had been suggested by one of the staff nurses, inquiring after my after-care treatment.

September 25th

At 7.10 a.m. I received a shock from the senior night nurse: 'You are going home today then, Percy?' she said. Straightaway I said, 'There must be a mistake for Mr Mac said Wednesday,' continuing, 'Well if that's so, I'd better get myself sorted out.' After breakfast, when the usual necessities were out of the way, and I'd had a quick read of the paper, one of the staff nurses on duty came in, so I told her, after she confirmed that I really was going home today, that I was pretty sure it was a mistake, and probably written down wrongly while all the kafuffle over the missing keys was going on. It was not long before I received a visit from the sister on duty, who had received my message. She asked, 'Will you stop another day?—as the insurance have no worries about your situation.' As I felt that I had made good progress, would do my walking exercises and have a general ability to cope with the problems that I knew would arise, I said ta-ta to those patients who had come in with me nearly twenty days ago. One lady I said goodbye to had come in with me, had gone home but was now back in again, having put her hip out getting in her son's motor—she was in the ward above now.

I went down to credit control to pay my accounts—I thought, after the amount of time spent here, the telephone bill would be astronomical—in a very happy state. I enjoyed my lunch at 12.00, ordered my taxi, collected my tablets from Pharmacy and after saying goodbye to several of the staff, I duly arrived home at 147, thinking that would be the last time I visited Holly House Hospital for some time.

I will only relate briefly the daily events that concerned my knee not improving after such major surgery on my left leg, and how it caused me so much concern through the following weeks. All the time I thought it was only a temporary hitch, that is until I was called back into hospital in November.

September 26th

I had a shocking night for, now I had been released from Holly House Hospital, I could no longer have the sleeping tablets that I'd so looked forward to. It was not long before I realised that I had left my glasses at the hospital and popping across to my neighbour Bert, asked him if he would be so kind as to pick them up for me when he was passing. Before the morning was over I had them returned to me. One of the first jobs I found that was going to be a regular one was the changing of the dressing each morning. I have made this statement in my diary—'Be glad when it stops oozing all this muck.' Later on I had to change the dressing. Blood coming through now.

September 27th

Up at 6.30 after having had a bad night and taking PK at 1.30

a.m. Straightaway I did some exercises on the bed with the leg still in its dressing at this stage, as I was told that it was important not to bend it if I want it to heal—important advice from the Holly House Hospital physio. In the afternoon, I had a telephone call from my old pal in Somerset to tell me he should have had an appointment at his hospital in Bristol, but at the last minute it had to be cancelled owing to emergency patients.

September 28th

Shocking night—took a couple of painkillers at 00.30 a.m. However I was up at 6.45 a.m. doing some exercises sitting on the table, which I now found to be more comfortable than lying on the bed. Changed the dressing, which appeared to be not quite so mucky, I was glad a friend of mine had given me several spare dressings when I arrived home on Tuesday for they were helping the cause no end.

September 29th

Had a better night for just before I went to bed I took some PK at 23.45. Up at 7.00 a.m. It's pouring with rain outside— and it's a sure thing that your body aches are in tune with the weather, for the whole of my leg is aching all the time, so I went and lay on the bed until nearly 10.00 a.m. During the rest of the day, I did some exercises almost every hour, after I had done some shopping.

Sunday, September 30th

I had a shocking night—even though I had taken a couple of PK before I went to bed at 12.00, the knee seems to be very hot. After my exercises on the bed and table, I changed the dressing, lots of muck in the old one. When I came back from collecting the newspaper, I did more exercises on the table and again at 14.00.

October 1st

Another bad night—seems as if the PK only works for a few hours. It's just a nagging pain which is there all the time. As the pain had not got any better after I had had my breakfast I decided to ring the district nurse at 9.40 a.m. Yes, she had a cancellation at 10.30.a.m. When my name was called and after the nurse had had a look at it she called in my GP, Dr Wong, who said, 'Yes, it does look nasty, take a swab; put a new dressing on and then get some more dressings for him on prescription.'

'Many thanks,' I said. The visit had helped my frame of mind no end—a relief to have the professional eye looking over the now pitiful knee. An appointment was made to see the nurse the following Friday afternoon at approximately 14.00. I did some exercises—and later in the early evening I did some more.

October 2nd

Bad night again—had taken my two tablets just before bedtime. At 7.15 a.m. I had done some exercises, also changed my dressing—it was the same sort of Micropore tape that the Holly House Hospital had used for me. According to the box there is 25mm by 5mm, so at the rate I use it I'll soon run out—no, don't get me wrong, I'm not one to waste anything, it's just that I perhaps use a bit more, for I have to let the knee in question bend—which I might add straightaway has not improved much on the ninety-five degrees that I had reached in Holly House Hospital. Later in the day I did some more exercises—also changed the dressing to find that the oozing was better as well—much less—as I have marked up.

Wednesday, October 3rd

I had a better night for I had taken my PK a bit later—in fact at 1.45. As I take about eight during the day (this is the amount to take in the twenty-four hours) I have to remember that I have already started my quota. By 6.30.a.m. I had completed bed and table exercises, and by 7.15 a.m. I had changed my dressing. I collected the morning paper, completed quite a bit of washing, for it was a nice bright dry start and I had decided to attack some washing which had been waiting to surface for some time. I completed this task with the washing line filled up from end to end. After I had done some more exercises—the time no later than 10.00 a.m.—I lay on the bed, knackered. 14.00, I decided to try and get the knee more mobile for I had an appointment with Mr Mac in the evening—so I completed more table and bed exercises. A friend of mine along the road came and picked me up—and dropped me off at Holly House Hospital. It appeared he was running behind his schedule so it was not until an hour later that I saw him. He had a good look at it: 'Looks fine, still swollen but give it time.' I told him that the surgery had taken a swab, and also given me a few dressings. The Outpatients' staff nurse put another dressing on, the material used being very similar to the surgery's. I was thankful for whatever was used since it was a source of a lot of comfort to me. 'I'll see you next Wednesday,' Mr Mac said.

October 4th

Shocking night again—I had taken my PK before I went to

bed at 11.45. At 3.10 a.m. I heard a loud bang which I am positive woke me up and from then onwards I could not get back to sleep. By 7.14 a.m. I had completed exercises and also changed my dressing. It's just a tiny hole now where the oozing is coming from and does not appear to want to heal up. 14.00, I did some more exercises on bed and table and as there was quite a bit of leaking from the old dressing decided to put another new one on—this after a good clean-up operation.

During the day I found a cat that had been run over and gave it a decent burial, though on making inquiries to my near neighbours as to whom it might have belonged to (for I know how much pain is involved when a treasured animal and friend disappears—the ache is unimaginable), nobody seemed to have seen a jet-black cat. Whilst I have only lived here a few years most of my neighbours seemed to be the sympathetic types I had been happy to find all my life. I had a painful evening to go through before I packed off to bed.

October 5th

I had taken a PK just before I went to bed at 23.45—made little difference for I could not sleep, so I had a rough night.

Up at 7.00 a.m. Exercises, bed and table. Then after breakfast—more exercises—bed and table for I thought to myself I must get the swelling down, which never seemed to reduce from one morning to another. I had made an appointment at my local GP's surgery for 10.30 a.m. I was in the surgery waiting for the nurse after walking down to the Drive, one of the local clinics in the district. The nurse very quickly attended to my dressing and, as the result from the swab had still not arrived, she phoned their lab who gave her the result which confirmed my own thoughts—that the bug was still very active. She spoke to Dr Wong who gave her a new prescription for me—a course of antibiotics, four to be taken at intervals over the twenty-four hours. I caught the bus back home for I was still worried in case any difficulties arose that needed urgent attention. What if the dressing needed changing? And there were hills all round coming away from the surgery! However, when I got back home I did some exercises which seemed to be quite comfortable. It was just after I had had my evening meal that I received a knock on the door. A young couple stood there introducing themselves, saying, 'We understand that you have found a cat.' I said, 'Come in.'

They were clutching a photo which was of the black cat I had found yesterday. Asking me, 'Is this the cat you found yesterday, Percy?' without hesitation I replied, 'Yes, I'm afraid so. I bet you were mighty proud of him.' 'Yes, we were, he was only two years old, named Charlie.' After I had assured them that he was now being well looked after in his animal kingdom, they went away knowing the whereabouts of their precious cat Charlie. I don't mind admitting that I also felt comfortable knowing that the couple knew their four-footed friend was now in his happy hunting ground.

However, when it was time to take my last tablets for the day I was glad the end of the day had arrived because I was putting up with a muddled head since I'd visited the surgery. It might have been the flu jab I had whilst I was there. Dr Wong had also suggested that I stop the Voltarol.

October 6th

Bad night again, mind you, as it was Saturday I treated myself to an extra hour in bed.

As I do not want to keep on repeating what occurred on a daily basis from this date until I was called back into Holly

House Hospital, I'll be as brief as possible—how my knee was subject to dressings, exercises, bad nights and progress.

October 10th

Saw Mr Mac, he seems unhappy with the swelling but says, 'We'll put a new dressing on and come and see me in a fortnight's time.' Nurse duly obliged with new dressing.

October 12th

Visit to district nurse in surgery; she had a look and changed the dressing I had put on some three hours earlier.

October 24th

Saw Mr Mac at 15.00: he seems very pleased with the new knee replacement after I had had another x-ray taken. It seems to be healing now.

October 25th

I had an appointment with the nurse at the surgery, told her that I had seen the big chief yesterday who was pleased with its progress: 'Yes, it's healing nicely.' Since the healing has now started—it seemed as if a whole weight has been lifted from my shoulders for I attacked all my daily chores with renewed gusto—the front garden now looks quite respectable.

November 3rd

I had a shocking night; there is a lot of swelling still around the repaired knee—in fact the whole knee is as big again as the other one. I was unprepared for this, for I have now used all the ice cubes from the fridge and so must use the next best thing for a cold poultice—and that's one pound of sausages and a piece of fish. At 8.00 a.m. I rang the surgery who told me they did not open until 9.00 a.m. I went and booked in to see the emergency doctor on duty who looked at it and said, 'Whew!' after gently feeling round the carbuncle shape that was now in front of both of us. He asked me what pills I had been taking after my operation and I also told him the daily dosage. 'The one I'm going to give you to take is twice a day—that should clear up the infection.' I took the pill as soon as I got back home, but can truthfully say I did not feel at all well for the rest of the day.

22.45—I thought I would leave it as late as possible before removing, tidying up, and replacing the dressing—I took everything off, covered up the carbuncle with a small dressing, making sure that no foreign bodies could make an entry, and fixed it all with Micropore, I then rubbed in Algersol, an old faithful of mine—around the painful parts of the swelling. It was when I was removing this lot of protection that in turn I lifted the scab. This was certainly not what I expected. It was as if I had turned a tap on: white-brown liquid started oozing out and running down my leg. I grabbed a tissue, hobbled into the kitchen, found a couple of boxes of tissues, returned to the living room, sat down for what seemed ages, while I waited for it to stop pumping out this vile stuff. Nearly two empty boxes later and it's almost midnight once I've tidied up the carpet and other places where I just could not prevent the discharge from spilling. I put a new dressing on, covered it with a table cloth, tied it all up with microtape and went to bed.

November 4th

What a mess—it's been oozing all night. It's not only gone through the whole of my dressing and improvised doubling-up but through the sheet and onto the mattress and underlay too. I could have cried. I put a fresh dressing on, walked to get my newspaper, then had to change it as soon as I got back because it had gone right through to my trousers. So what I did then was change from my trousers to a pair of shorts which served the purpose adequately. For the rest of the day I kept quiet—it might have been because I put two dressings lower down the leg as well. I typed a letter to Mr Mac telling him of the situation I had found myself in the night before. I considered afterwards—as I am a very much below average patient, these setbacks are to be expected. He must be fed up, but, like I stated in the letter, it would have been nice if I could have been prepared for this mini-explosion. One of the neighbours who saw me just as I was putting some washing out nearly fainted when she saw the wound and the disturbance it had caused to nearby tissues. For the rest of the day it continued to ooze; I cannot recall how many dressings I replaced, but I know I was mighty glad when it was time for bed, hoping that I was not going to have another night like last night—but I was well prepared this time for not only had I taken the same precautions as the previous night but had found one of the big bath towels and placed it directly under my body, stretched right across the bed.

Monday, November 5th

I was up at 7.00 a.m. According to the state of the dressing there had been a fair bit of discharge, so I tidied it up and replaced it with a new one, then went out and got my paper.

At 9.00 I rang the surgery to see if the nurse would have a look and give me some advice. Yes—they can fit me in at 11.10 a.m. On my way I delivered the letter I had typed for Mr Mac at Holly House Hospital for him to browse over. The nurse was making good progress with her patients as she saw me at 11.00. As Dr Wong was on duty he was brought in to give an opinion—telling him of the surprise I had just before 23.00 last Saturday night and the muck that I was concealing around my knee joint. 'Certainly,' he said, 'you have an infection.' He wanted another swab taken to see if the tablets I was now taking were efficient—also telling the nurse to try using some seaweed to plug the hole in the wound. This of course was a soul-destroying piece of flesh to look at, for it appeared bottomless when a probe was placed inside. It was a good job I was of good healthy stock and knew how to skin and gut a rabbit, for many a person would by this time have wanted some smelling salts to bring them back to the land of the conscious. After a good tidying-up job had been accomplished, the nurse seemed to be confident that using the seaweed as a plug would not only heal it quickly but also make it more comfortable for me. Then, finally, with a new liniment and dressing in place, I left with a much more contented mind than the disturbed one I had arrived with. For the rest of the day I carried out my usual chores and did not even interfere with dressings any more. Before I went to bed I took my last allocation of painkillers and my usual measures for protecting the sheets. I had noticed that some of the muck had got onto the top sheet, but rather than change them both, I put on a clean one to lie on, then turned round the top stained one so it was now at the bottom of the bed and on the other side; it worked a treat.

November 6th

Up at 6.00 a.m. I have recorded good luck!! Not much muck—had put another tea towel over the one already in place where I lay—fortunately I had not wriggled about much so the bed was okay. For the rest of the day, the knee kept on discharging at various times and in between using my typewriter, I had to stop, tidy it up with paper tissues and put a fresh dressing on according to the notes I have put down!!! My God!!!! There has been some rubbish come out today—in fact the last note of the day says I have used two boxes of tissues!!! At 22.45, I took the whole of the dressing off and replaced it with a completely new one—the amount that came off half-filled a carrier bag. I am going to try to keep it on all night.

November 7th

I had a comfortable night and as there was no discharge I kept the dressing on—for I was to see the district nurse this morning at 9.40 a.m. After I had had my breakfast I received a call from Mr Mac's secretary to say he wants to see me this afternoon. 'No, don't worry about an appointment, he will see you as soon as you come in.' So it certainly looked as if this was getting serious but at no time did I understand how serious the situation was getting. When I saw the nurse in due course, she appeared most concerned but cheered up immensely when I told her Mr McAuliffe was going to see me this afternoon; however, she tidied the knee up and replaced the old stained dressing with a clean one. Mr Mac saw me at 16.45. Straightaway he felt all the way round and down the knee in question and said, 'I want you to come into Holly House Hospital right away.' Then, making enquiries, he found that no beds were available anywhere in Holly House. 'Make arrangements to come in tomorrow at 10.00 a.m.' He added, 'I am going to cut you up again, I'm afraid, and give the whole lot a good clear out to cleanse your system.' I said, 'Surely not?' 'Yes,' he replied, nodding his head. So when I got back home—a round of telephone calls and cancellations because if it was going to be like the last time it was certainly going to be a fortnight at least.

November 8th

I was up at 6.20 a.m. for there was a lot for me to do. One good thing was that there wasn't any muck. By 7.00 a.m. I had been down to the paper shop and picked up the paper. What I have noticed is that I am certainly slowing up with my walking, doing my chores and the many etceteras. I have had strict orders that I must not eat anything after 8.00 a.m. so working it all out I would most likely be going down for the operation early in the afternoon, but then this was Thursday and already Mr Mac's plans for today had been allocated to patients who had perhaps been waiting months—so wait and see. I drove my motor up to my friend who lives next door to Holly House Hospital. I had previously asked permission to leave it in one of his garage spaces—knowing it was going to be safe. On arrival at Holly House Hospital, I was taken up to the second floor and allocated a room number—268. I had a few tests to make sure that I had not undergone too many changes from my last visit—just about six weeks ago. All the checks were made on the one machine—the ECG. I have a visit from the accounts department to inform me that everything is okay to go ahead, thus confirming what I already knew, since I had been in touch with my insurers by phone advising that this was an ongoing problem from the operation I had back in September. I'd had a phone call back from the company—

'Yes, it's all in order to have another operation.' Mr Dodd arrives at 13.00. In fact he almost followed Mr Mac in who'd had me sign on the dotted, and marked up the leg in question. Mr Dodd says that I can have a cuppa, as there could be a delay. Yes, there sure was a delay of several hours. I did not go down to theatre until 21.00 hours. This was to make sure that the theatre was germ-free—as I must not get another infection—however, I was not down there too long, back in the room at 22.15 hours. I had all the usual attachments fixed to me plus one of the nurses with me for most of the night. I dare say it was on one of the few occasions that she was not with me that I must have done some joggling about so that I managed to upset the bottle that scavenges and collects rubbish so that it discharged straight onto the lower sheet.

November 9th

Change of sheets before trolley came round—and then ready for the early morning cuppa at 7.15. Everything going according to plan. I have a visit from the physiotherapist after breakfast. I was sitting out in the armchair but after this visit I was told to get back into bed. So stayed the rest of the day doing a few exercises, enjoying all the food that was sent in to me. As I have no monkey pole attached to the bed I am pretty insistent that someone locate one for me—it's an L-shaped piece of two-inch tubular iron which is connected to the bed. The other part of the L is just over your head with a strap attached so you can adjust the height—then with this strap you can lever yourself around the bed, make movements up or down the bed or from side to side. Eventually one was found for me, which made me feel more comfortable.

The dinner, when it arrived was unfortunately, not what I thought I had ordered; it had substantial amounts of red spices with it, which I cannot stand at any price—only just the faintest smell puts me off.

November 10th

I have marked down 'not a bad night', so, as far as I was concerned, this was one when I slept for most of the night, with no doubt the SPs doing their job.

The duties all completed, the physio arrives just before 10.00 a.m.; she decides that all I have to do is some exercises on the bed, and as she was on duty again in the afternoon, this was the same procedure then.

I enjoyed all the chef had provided at 12.15 hours, leaving reasonably clean plates.

Mr Mac came in to see me just before England kicked off against Sweden; he tells me that the drain attached to the wound can come out now, and tells the Staff Nurse taking those notes that he has put stitches in, instead of staples. No, he has not gone so low this time with his cutting, as he thought it unnecessary. Yes, get out of bed and exercise—this is all beneficial to the improvement of the knee.'

I have had an African nurse looking after me since the change-over in the afternoon, and when she came in soon after Mr Mac had completed his rounds, I had already been out to the toilet ,and had a wash, shave, etc.

She was surprised when I passed on this information, for she had been told, 'He must not get out of bed!' More surprises were in store for her, for I got out of the bed and walked across to the door! I said to her, 'You must be passing on some of your magic,' for I had heard that she was from one of the tribal regions.

Again I don't suppose she understood , though she might have received confirmation from the staff nurse earlier that it was all right for the patient in Room 268 to exercise.

Later I had a cup of hot chocolate and later still PK.

Sunday Nov 11th

I have marked up not a bad night. I don't know why because not only is my chest playing up (it's the cold I came in with, which is now developing into a bronchial one I am sure) but the bed—what a mess! It's been discharging for a lot of the night, so the night nurse changes the dressing, where it has oozed through, and, though only a tiny stain on the sheet, those changed too to make everywhere all wholesome again.

Looking at the areas disturbed, it looks as if the problem piece is going to be awkward again in healing for it's almost in the identical place as the area that previously gave us all a lot of worry. When the physio arrived I was out of bed waiting for her; exercises for a start—then a walk down the corridor and a walk up and down the staircase. This was most peculiar for I got the sequence wrong for doing this.. Good leg—stick—bad leg; but it was not long after I had come up for the second time that I got the hang of it again. Back in Room 268 I considered that it was about time that I sent a decent letter off to the insurance company—so I got stuck into that for the rest of the afternoon and completed it. The dressing has started to weep through but it does not seem to be too bad. Before I went to sleep I had asked for a sleeping tablet: 'No, not until the doctor on duty has authorised it.'

November 12th

Had a bad night, but when I told her I'd had a rough night the night nurse said that each time she came in to see how I was I was fast asleep. I must remember to ask if I can have another try for a sleeping tablet tonight. She then said, 'You do know that the sleeping tablet was brought to you by the night nurse on duty and as you were asleep at the time she did not want to wake you.' What could I say?—only one thing, 'Oh let's forget about it, shall we? Must be me!!!' Can't believe I said this. A visit from the physio, doing just bed exercises. I also had a visit from one of Mr Mac's secretaries. I had asked her, as it was rather an important letter to the insurance company, could she say if it was drafted appropriately. 'Yes, it reads fine,' she said after reading the contents. Ate all of my lunch which included ham, eggs and chips, with one of the fruit desserts that I came to enjoy tremendously, because they had such a variety of assorted items on the plate. 14.30 hours staff nurse came in with a nebuliser to help my breathing for my chest had not improved a lot. This certainly made a big difference to my lungs and chest. Mr Mac called in to see how I was getting on, removing the dressing straightaway—and am sure he was happy with what he saw for he said, 'I'll have another look at it tomorrow, then you can go home on Wednesday.' I asked, 'Do you think that it will be all right for travelling on?' His reply: 'Yes,' he nodded, telling the staff, 'The lower stitches can come out now.' This was accomplished without any difficulty within ten minutes of his leaving; cleaned and just a dressing to cover the top part of the knee, where the wound was till discharging. Where those fibre stitches were it did look a rough job—but when I mentioned this on one occasion to Mr Mac he laughed and said, 'Looks fine to me.' What I don't consider before I say something like this is the fact that the skin has been disturbed before—thus making it difficult for the healing to take place. What I do know is that Mr Mac is very patient with me and does not attempt to further my conversation with him, just a nod and a grin. I dare say he says in his own mind, 'We have a right one here!'

At 23.00 hours I had a sleeping tablet and PK before I went off to sleep.

November 13th

6.40 a.m. The night nurse taking my observations tells me that my blood pressure is up. She has a look at the dressing. We both agree that it looks all right, then at 7.05 a.m. I had turned over to find that there wasn't half a mess in the bed where the wound had been discharging through the night. I could have cried. Something that I tried not to do whilst I was in hospital was press the bell for attention, but I did this right away. Within a second the staff nurse had arrived, and seeing the bed and mess said, 'I'm glad that you've told me, for the night sister was just finalising her notes and reporting that you were OK.'

Everything changed, clean and tidy within ten minutes. A swab had been already taken yesterday, and was awaiting the result from the lab! Now another one!! Is this for another bug, or is it the same one that's tormenting me? l don't know!! Later in the morning I am told to take two new tablets four times a day. Piece of fish for lunch, second lot of tablets 13.30 hours.

Here's a strange coincidence: I was watching Sky News on the television, and reading the *Cricketer*—a monthly magazine; the article I was reading concerned a well-known cricketer of the 1930s, '40s, and '50s, named Eddie Paynter. He was one of the England test team in the Body-Line series of 1932-33 and had started the Fourth Test but was laid low in a private hospital in Brisbane after suffering slight sunstroke and tonsillitis, following the first day's play. England were not faring too well in reply to Australia's total of 340. So word was sent to him from Douglas Jardine the England Captain via Bill Voce, saying, 'How about those fellows who marched to Kandahar with the fever on them?' This apparently acted like a tonic to Eddie, who immediately discharged himself, went out next day and played a magnificent innings of 83!!! Then he scored 14 not out in the second innings, England winning by 6 wickets.

And here I am watching the Sky News, telling me that the North Alliance Troops are now marching on Kandahar!

19.00 hours: I take more tablets; they're all serving a purpose to help clear my system of its impurities. Each time the old dressing is taken off and replaced with a new one, I look at the stitches on either side and wonder how it will look eventually.

It was not long after I was thinking about this that Mr Mac arrives with sister and a nurse, both taking notes. He helps to remove the dressing, looking at it, says, 'I'll pop in tomorrow to see if the weeping has improved.' It was at this stage when we were all looking at the wound and stitches that I casually mentioned to him—about one part in the middle where the stitches did not appear to be in alignment with those on the other side, asking, 'Will this make any difference at some later stage?' Listening to this outburst from me, they all three had a good laugh with Mr Mac replying, 'Nothing to worry about at all, will take a little longer to heal that's all.'

But I'd had to ask, not to hurt anyone's feeling but just to release pressure that builds up if I see something out of place and incorrect. I did learn a lot from this little explosion and it has since been drummed into me that the skin, after a wound has been made and the initial healing has taken place, tends to have some more fragile parts around some bits of the cut than others, and it is difficult to get the threads to find a firm foundation, hence the reason why it did not look like a job well done. Mind you—it all depends on how the surgeon likes to perform his task, for as I walked round chatting I noticed how stitches are done quite differently by other surgeons and equally the end product turns out to be a splendid repair in most instances I have seen.

Later, all the tablets were taken on time and at 23.30 hrs I have the last of the day's quota of antibiotics.

November 14th

Evidently it's still leaking as there is a patch on the bed, but nothing like as big as other mornings. When the night nurse had taken my observations, I asked her how my blood pressure was, and she told me that it seemed all right today. By 9.00 a.m. I had done all my ablutions and the sheets had been changed.

10 a.m. Another staff nurse comes in to change my dressing. This had been on for about three hours, not much had come through but this staff nurse did something that I have almost willed the other staff and nurses to do—give the whole area around the aperture a good squeeze. When she did this, my! Wasn't there some muck come out! Telling her that all the staff on duty have different methods and after looking down into the cavity I was surprised how deep it was. It made sense to me that by freeing all the pus and muck this would help the internals to heal and improve more quickly!!!! Or so I thought!!!!

At 17.00 hrs. Mr Mac comes in and without looking at anything (no doubt—been informed of my situation by the sister) just said, 'We'll give it another day.' I said, 'It's been quite painful today.' He replied, 'You have to be patient.' For the rest of the day, I did my exercises and walked along to the other wings—down the lift onto the first floor, walk round chatting to those patients whom I had got to know after my freedom from 268 had begun. As usual I asked after their health and likewise they after mine, each comparing and inquiring about what sort of operations had been carried out. Mostly it seemed that knee replacements like mine would be out in just about a fortnight with the stitches being removed about a day or so prior to release, again circumstances permitting.

I made an important phone call to say could one of my pals pick up some shopping for me as I was confident I would be home on Friday.

Last thing—tablets and turned the telly off.

November 15th

There has been some discharge during the night so the night nurse has changed the sheets before the day staff have taken over. Mind you, this does not really matter because it is usual for the day shift nurses to change everyone's bedlinen even if, as in some of my own instances, it might well have been on only ten minutes. Off it all comes and is replaced with another clean set. I was sure I was going to go home before the weekend and confident that I could cope with the conditions prevailing. However, as there was more discharge during the morning, and when Mr Mac called in later he said, 'Give it a few more days,' I realised that it would be useless to go home. I should have had to be loaded down with new sterile dressings, microtape, etc. etc.

I now had to phone everyone I had phoned before to say that I was not coming home until after the weekend now. One call was important though, because now I was stuck here again, I could not read my post at home, so a good pal went and collected the keys from a neighbour, picked up all the post and brought it up to Holly House Hospital for me to read and digest; this duly arrived in the afternoon.

For the rest of the day—usual exercises, bed and walking, but no stair work, as it seemed it was most important for the wound to heal. Another call I nearly forgot was to the editor of our parish news, whom I had told I would be home on Saturday. We had to rearrange the venue for meeting to Holly House Hospital, that is, if it was convenient to her. When I got in touch with her—'No problem,' she said, 'see you on Saturday.' One of my last notes I have recorded for today is: 'I have been worn out today.'

November 16th

Not a bad night; it has leaked a bit during the night and I will be interested to know if any healing has taken place when the dressing is taken off. I'd had a good night sleep-wise.

After breakfast and all regular duties accomplished, I had a walk. Then nurse changed the dressing. It appears to be still oozing a little!!!! While it's doing this it certainly will not heal, which is giving great concern over its unwillingness to join up and make everyone happy, including yours truly.

I thought it was going to be a day whereby the tide was turning in my favour. However, this was not to be. I don't know why the fates that be were treating me this way, because I had been quietly busy, doing no harm! Busy with pen and paper when I was not fulfilling other obligations. I had just enjoyed my dinner when Mr Mac called in whilst I was sitting in the armchair beside the bed. The staff came round with him taking notes whilst he was reading up my itinerary. He then said after examining the gungy muck that was now leaking from it, 'We'll give it a few more days.'

It was when I went to get back onto the bed that the pocket of blood, which had been collecting in a cell somewhere, decided to break out. There was then a big disturbance for a few minutes, for it just would not stop, according to my diary. It was coming out as if I was a stuck pig. In about ten minutes all was back to normal again, with myself a few millilitres lighter, with clean sheets and a clean dressing. I wondered what tomorrow was going to bring. What I did mark up during this mini-panic—one of the nurses liked my voice. It had a certain brogue which her daughter, she knew, would be thrilled with. Could she bring her round and have a chat with me? And there's me telling people before I have met them by post or whatever—you will have to accept the voice, it's what I was born with.

Last remark for the day—knackered!

November 17th

Not a bad night considering. 7.10 a.m. cuppa, 8.30 a.m. breakfast, after wash and brush-up, went for a walk. Then a new dressing put on after old one has been discarded and this time, as instructed, I had bandages as well as dressings attached and finished off with Microtape. 12.00—Mr Mac called in to see about progress, looks at the wad of bandage and says, 'We'll see what it's like on Monday.' 12.30: lunch arrives—salad with ham and other delicacies laid out on lettuce leaves. My, how this Sunday chef is never outdone by the chefs who supply our meals during weekdays. Sometimes I feel it's unkind to interfere with the decoration. However this time justice was done—I ate the lot. Then my visitor arrived in the afternoon and left a cake for me!!!! Whew!!!!

November 18th

Not a bad night, which means I slept reasonably well with very little wriggling about. Cuppa at 7.00 a.m. Yes, the weekend waitresses are on the ball, just like the weekday girls.

The dressing has not been touched so far. This was after I had had my breakfast, sheets changed and gone for a walk and back in the room again. By 9.30 a.m. the staff in charge came and tidied it up and there was very little weeping.

As I am not having much physio done—only just bed exercises and walking, the idea being to make sure that healing takes place first, during the course of the morning it seemed quite painful.

12.00—I'll just mention what I had for lunch, as I have marked it down as a bit special—roast pork, cauliflower, Brussels, boiled potatoes, and roast ones, apple sauce, dessert rhubarb and custard. When my readings were done later, the blood pressure was up and my knee was also still painful.

November 19th

Twelfth day since the operation. I have a good night, with breakfast arriving at 8.20 a.m. When the dressing came off at 9.30 a.m., it was reasonably dry, with very little discharge. By that time I had done some exercises on the staircase. In fact, five times up and down, so I was pleased that the exercising had put a certain amount of pressure on the knee without doing too much damage. Mind you, it was pretty painful.

Mr Mac came along, did not look at his work, just said, 'We'll have a look tomorrow.'

Through the day I had several walkabouts, also inquiring after various patients' health. I also had a visit from the accounts lady, who informs me that my insurance company want an update on my progress, which she has given them. All in order.

November 20th

At 6.40 a.m. I have had all the vitals done, also a cuppa at 7.15 a.m., breakfast completed by 8.30 a.m. As the dressing looks dry, it's agreed to leave it until Mr Mac arrives. However,

I walked up and down the staircase a few times. 16.15 hrs, Mr Mac arrives, the dressing is uncovered after some thirty hours. It's dry, and it's certainly showing more home-going potential. He says, 'We will take the stitches out on Thursday, then see how it goes.' I told him, 'I am concerned about the knee bending for it's some time since I was on the machine. I feel it's going backwards.' I mentioned that I had seen the physiotherapist this morning. 'Yes,' he said, 'and so have I. Don't worry about the bending, let's get it healed.'

Later, after I had had my dinner and made a few phone calls, one of the nurses came in with a bottle of tablets to take home with me. They had been collected from the pharmacy, for they understood that I was going home. So I politely told her to take them back because nobody was going home from Room 268 until the stitches are taken out.

November 21st

Not a bad night. I am sure I slept right through until 5.00 a.m. So am confident that at long last, when I can sleep without any interruption that things are going my way at last. (How wrong could I be!)

All tasks and duties completed by 8.45 a.m. I then went for a walk on stairs and down corridors whilst nurse changed the sheets back in Room 268. The staff comes in, changes dressings. Looking good, though swollen.

I take a walk down to Credit Control to find out how my telephone bill, amongst other items, is progressing. She said she would check it all out and let me know. I had made several long-distance calls so I knew it was going to be a lot more than my usual home bill. Not long before 13.10 hours I had a call to say that everything is almost complete and will be ready for my discharge tomorrow. So again someone has jumped the gun and discharged me before it has been confirmed by Mr Mac himself. 'That's news to me,' I said.

I did some more staircase work in the afternoon and evening, with the pain much more tolerable. Last thing pills—PK and ST. Thankfully my chest has been okay now for three or four days. So those pills have been given the heave.

November 22nd

Not a bad night. It seems to have been weeping just a little. There was also a first experience after I had my early morning cuppa. I listened for the breakfast trolley. Certainly it came and then silence. Returned back to headquarters without paying a visit to me! By 8.30 a.m. I made inquiries as to my breakfast and it was then realised that they had forgotten me. I will say that Thursday is a day when this sort of thing can easily occur because it's the busiest day of the week with all the theatres working from as early as 7.30 a.m. 'Sorry about this, Percy!!!' I then went for a walk, keeping out of the way of traffic and only moving about when it was reasonably sensible to do so. By 10.30 a.m. the stitches had been removed and a new dressing had been put on. As the corridor was quiet outside, I had another walk, seemed quite comfortable. 12.20 a.m. Mr Mac came in, had a look at the wound which was now weeping just a little, said, 'You can go home this afternoon or tomorrow.'

I said, 'I would prefer tomorrow for it will give me a chance to organise myself for home duties if that's all right?'

'Yes, fine,' he says. For the rest of the day I was phoning various people to say that I will be coming out tomorrow. It's surprising the amount of people who were interested in me and my health. Other duties which were important were my exercises, up and down the staircase. It seems pretty painful to bend, even now the stitches are out but, thinking back, it's some time since I had been on the CPM so this no doubt was one of the reasons why it was painful and stiff. 20.30 hours—I have my final dressing put on. This will be the third one today. During the day I had a visit from the admin department to ask me how everything is and can I cope when I arrive back home? 'Yes of course I can,' said I, thinking that I was now on the road to recovery. Pills and tablets and dressings all taken care of as well.

November 23rd

Sixteenth day. Not a bad night. After I had finished early morning cuppa, breakfast, quick read of newspaper, I went and had a shower. Obviously the dressing got soaked but on removing it I found it had been leaking, but it appeared to have dried up when I had completed my towelling down. In any case I started changing into my going-home clothes; the staff nurse comes in whilst I am preparing and, seeing that the wound is leaking not only muck but also blood as well, puts a fresh dressing on. 11.00—I went and said ta-ta to a few people and by 11.45 a.m. I was back at home. My good Samaritan arrived with all the shopping that I had asked for and we were soon partaking of a nice cuppa. By 17.00 hours I had changed another dressing—seems the same muck is coming through. I also am now back on my usual pills including those I have to take whilst I still have pills to clear up the infection—which I presume I still have.

November 24th

Now back home, there is no one to make or bring me an early morning cuppa. I did not have a bad night. I made sure about leakage for I had placed a towel over the bottom sheet, because

I was not in a position to keep changing sheets every time one or the other got soiled. I found it had leaked a little, so it was no problem to wash out the towel later. I put on another clean dressing, after tidying up the wound which I convinced myself seemed heaps better. Several jobs around I found, like clearing gullies (drain) blocked with leaves. Had a few visitors during the day all wanting to know if I was going to be all right this time. I told them to wait and see. Most wanted to know what had been done the second time. All I could tell them was what I'd been told—that I had been cut open again, in the same place and had what is termed 'a good wash-out', which has now cleared my system and I was now waiting to heal up.

November 25th

Had a walk down to get the morning paper. The knee aches like hell. Most of the day I tried to rest it as much as possible but with visitors, it's getting up making a cuppa, sitting down, getting up, etc. etc. 17.00 hours—cooked my main meal for the day—fried fish, mash, cabbage and an apple. When I had eaten this, had a wash and shave, I then changed the dressing which had a fair amount of discharge appearing, resting through the rest of the evening until I put a fresh one on at 23.30 hours; at this time just a little weeping.

November 26th

I have marked up a terrible night. During the night I have tried to keep the leg reasonably level, for I have found that if I can keep on one side without turning over, this not only helps the pain, but also keeps the muck from activating itself. Even then, I have hardly slept at all. I have decided not to go for the newspaper because this only aggravates it, and makes it flare up. This did not make much difference because as soon as I had got up and prepared my breakfast and completed my other chores, it started discharging again—another clean dressing used. Monday today and my Mrs Mopp arrived at 11.00 to do some tidying up for me and a bit of polishing.

Rested for the rest of the day until cooking started again. I enjoyed the fish I had prepared, this time boiled with some parsley sauce (from out of the garden). I also receive a big parcel which gives me more homework to attend to. This together with phone calls, both in and out going kept me busy for the rest of the day. At 23.30 hours, I change the dressing. Although the discharge is improving, there is still a lot of blood and pus.

November 27th

Rough night again. When I say rough night again, I mean just that, for my bedclothes are invariably in total disarray, with me concerned as to what I should do, lay there, get up, walk about, make a cuppa? And now my waterworks are playing up as well. Then I keep reminding myself of others and count that I am one of the lucky ones. I decide to keep the dressing on, though some blood had appeared during the night, but it's not bad.

What has occurred during the night is a very sharp frost which is giving us a very clear and bright morning. Toast for breakfast, then a round of chores including typing a letter to a very important person who is beginning to take over my life—my publisher!!!! By 13.30 hours, after I had walked to the post box and posted the letters, it started to rain. Phone calls rest of day among some other jobs, then bedtime at 23.30. I kept the dressing on, but took a couple of painkillers.

November 28th

Shocking night. It looks as if the wound is holding this morning so decide to leave the dressing on. It's 8.00 a.m. and have again decided not to go for paper, so I am going to rest it as much as I can. At 17.00 hours I was preparing to do my cooking and had not interfered with the dressing all day when, looking down at my leg, I felt something that I thought was a dozy fly walking about. !!!!NOT SO!!!! BLOOD AND PUS running down my leg and it just would not stop. Fortunately I had got a good supply of tissues in, so grabbing one of the boxes, I used most of them up, then finding a good crepe bandage I wrapped this round the whole leg. The ooze had run into the sock as well, so I had to change my socks as well as tidying up the mess lying about. Just completed this duty—knock on door, my neighbour from along the road came to see how I was. 'Cor blimey, Perc. It ain't half swollen,' he said on seeing the bandage. 'No,' I replied, 'you should have come a little while ago when I had a big problem with it bursting out,' and I showed him the carrier with the discarded tissues.

In the afternoon I was doing exercises whilst lying on the settee when I thought I might just as well lie on the bed and do some quads contractions. This is an old practice to strengthen your leg and thigh muscles. Also pushing upwards and outwards with leg movements. This from side to side. I suppose total time about ten minutes, certainly no longer.

At 19.00 hours after I had had a wash and brush-up, I knew by the feel of how I was walking that I must change the dressing which I attended to straightaway. It was a right mess with blood oozing out as well as muck. I had now convinced myself that if the stitches had been put in correctly with the steel ones, like the first operation, none of this would have occurred. By this time I was wise to what may follow. I found that by wrapping something like an old flannel below the knee with paper tissues bound round with the Micropore, this would absorb any of the muck running down my leg.

It was 23.40 hours when I took this lot off and placed the final dressing and tissues plus a towel as the last covering. There had been a fair amount of mess coming out during those few hours that had passed and I just wondered where it had all come from and how it is still finding its way out through the little hole.

I have finally recorded—'Dreading the night.'

November 29th

Not a bad night after all. Up at 8.00 a.m. Tidied up the mess and replaced it with clean dressings. As I realised that this was getting serious, the first thing after breakfast (three pieces of toast) I got the Sharp out and typed a letter to Mr Mac, started at 8.30, completed and put into an envelope by 9.15 a.m. I then contacted Holly House Hospital explaining what was happening. A call back within the hour to say make my way to Outpatients as soon as I can. Arriving at 10.30, I left the letter for Mr Mac's secretary to attend to. Going straight to Outpatients, the duty nurse immediately took a swab, after the RD had suggested this. He then phoned Mr Mac, who said he would call in to see me around 13.00 hours. When he arrived I told him what I had done yesterday, and asked if I had disrupted the healing process. 'I doubt that,' he said, continuing, 'See what the swab says. If it's positive that there is an infection, I shall have to cut you up again and find out if the infection is near the bone.'

'What! Cut me open again!!!' I gasped.

'I'm afraid so,' was his reply and he was gone.

Last thing at night I changed the dressing for a more substantial one including another fresh towel.

November 30th

I slept until 5.00 a.m. and was pretty sure that wriggling about has disturbed the wound, so by 6.30 a.m. I took the lot off to find a right mess. This appeared to be the same colour as the first discharge or to my eyes, it certainly appeared so. I was also finding it an improvement to wrap several layers of tissues around and over the fresh sterile dressings firmly tethered down with the Microtape.

I got up at 7.15 a.m. Did not bother going for a paper but I certainly missed it. Friday is normally a busy day, as I like to get myself organised for the weekend but today I felt really choked, thinking that I might have to go back into Holly House Hospital to be cut open again. Weather outside has not helped anybody's spirits neither. Through the day, it's been raining on and off since daybreak.

23.30 hours I took off the old dressing and replaced it with a new one. I had earlier in the day phoned Holly House Hospital Outpatients telling the sister in charge that I was finding it difficult to stop the wound from leaking. She suggested that I could only do as I had been doing, place a towel or something similar round the whole lot to soak up any discharge that might ooze through. Looking at what I had wrapped round my knee, I was confident that I had made a secure job.

December 1st

This was Saturday. A day that I always look forward to, not only in the summer months but winter ones as well. I did not have a bad night. I was moving about at 7.30 a.m. The old dressing had done a handsome job for though it had oozed through, none had got onto the bath towel I had now spread right across the bed. After breakfast I made myself respectable because I had an appointment with Mr Mac and Outpatients at 10 a.m. On arrival, the duty nurse took off all the old dressings, telling me that Mr Mac was delayed, so a temporary covering was placed over the wound and microtaped down. Whilst waiting, the waitresses looked after me with sandwiches and tea. On his appearance and following an examination in his consulting room, he told me the result of the swab which did not look good, and explained he is now going to put me on another course of tablets. In fact, two different sorts of antibiotics. These take me up to this coming Wednesday; then, if there is no improvement, he will bring me in, and cut down deeper to find the source of the infection. He then proceeded to write me out a prescription, took a hasty look and prescribed a few tablets, I thought I had sufficient money to pay for them; after all it was only a few days' treatment. On the way out I also collected more dressings from Outpatients. At the pharmacy I was presented with the account for the tablets, which worked out at nearly one pound per tablet.

This remark came out automatically, with no thought to anyone around. 'Who do you think I am!!!!!—Lord Rothschild!!!' I am sure the pharmacist did not understand me because I received a super smile. However, I found sufficient money to pay for one lot of tablets. I then decided to go home to Loughton, pick up some more funds, return and settle the account. On the way home, I passed my own GP's surgery, so called in to see if the emergency doctor could let me have a prescription for those special tablets. This was hard luck for they had closed at 11.00 a.m. So back home, pick up the necessary money, back to Holly House Hospital, pay up, pick up, saying to the pharmacist, 'I hope these are worthy of the time and money I have spent on them, for I am sure they are the costliest pills I have ever purchased!' I am sure you can understand how I was feeling for the disappointments were beginning to pile up. For as each new day was starting, a big worry was of course the arrangements to be made to travel with the England cricket supporters to see the three test matches against New Zealand. Time was certainly moving on to sort out company and travel options for February and March of next year—2002.

Last thing before I went to bed was change the dressing, having taken my last pills of the day, for I so much wanted another visit to Holly House Hospital to be only a pipe dream.

December 2nd

Up at 8.00 a.m. after a pretty good night. Dressing clean, bed—nothing had come through—in any case I took the old one off and changed it for a fresh one, making a good job with the Microtape. Through the day I kept busy doing various duties about the house, including some washing, later to find it had hardly dried out on the clothes line at all. Last thing at night I gave the dressing an inspection. Hardly any discharge and certainly there was nothing like so much pain, this after I had done a few exercises on the bed but nothing strenuous.

December 3rd

7.40 a.m. First job—changed dressing, nothing like as much discharge—but unfortunately the colour that is coming out, slightly bloody, is the same as other times in the past, this after I have given it a good squeeze. I went for a morning paper but took my time.

My Mrs Mopp arrived at 11.00 a.m. for a general tidy up

and to perform a duty I did not think I would ever ask of anyone and that was to store my dahlia tubers safely away for me in the cupboard under the upstairs flat's staircase.

Restful day with a few exercises, nothing that could harm the healing if and when it takes place.

Last pills after I had changed the dressing for the final time at 22.00 hours.

December 4th

Not a bad night. I must have made a good job of the dressing because it has stayed on all night, changing this just after I got up at 7.00 a.m. I went up to the churchyard later just to tidy up a few graves. After ten minutes I noticed that discharge had started to stain my trousers, so packed this up straightaway, went home and changed into my shorts, also changed the dressing, both blood and muck had come through so as I have described it—A BLOODY MESS!!!

Last thing—pills and fresh dressing before I turned in.

December 5th

Not a bad night. There has been no discharge. Is it stopping? However, I changed the dressing and made a good job of tape around the disturbed area for I had decided to leave the dressing on for I had to see Mr Mac this afternoon. Another assignment which I look forward to is how my Xmas cards have grown in quantity over the years, how a letter is always welcomed and trust that all mine are received in the same spirit. Anyhow I have located around forty, so this is a mammoth start, this will have to be done before long.

At 14.45 hours, nurse calls me in to see Mr Mac. The dressing comes off. He asks me about the discharge, which is now hardly showing at all, it's almost slowed down. He says, after thinking what next to do, 'We will give it until Saturday, with the same sort of treatment,' and reaches for his prescription pad!!!! I said, 'You have no objection if I collect them from my own doctor in the Clinic in the Drive, Mr Mac, do you?' 'No certainly not,' is his reply, continuing, 'What we will do is take a blood sample.' A new dressing was then put on, with an appointment made for the following Saturday at 15.50 hours; a swab was also taken. On the way back home, I called into the doctor's surgery where the reception girls are just as super as the ones in Holly House Hospital, so within a quarter of an hour I had picked up the prescription, taken it to a nearby chemist who duly obliged with more supplies.

Last thing—change of dressing, seemed clean at 22.00 hours.

December 6th

Pretty good night, there has been very little discharge!!!! So after all this time has a genuine heal started?

I was up at 7.15 a.m. as there was nothing to concern me with the dressing, I left it on and kept it on all day until I changed it just before I went to bed. During all this time, hardly anything had come out, it looked as if something was happening though—it was still swollen.

December 7th

Not a bad night. Dressing seemed okay, got up at 7.05 a.m. and took a steady walk for the paper, dry, frosty morning. The rest of the day, after breakfast I had quite a bit of paperwork to do especially accounts to settle, then a walk down to the post box with the completed letters.

Kept the dressing on for the rest of the day, when I changed it at about 23.00 hours, it had now been on for twenty-four hours so when I removed it, I expected to find problems but no, there had been just a little discharge. Soon all tidied up and a new dressing put in place.

December 8th

I had had my appointment moved from the afternoon to an early morning one for 10.30 a.m. to see Mr Mac. When I got up at 8.00 a.m. I mention that I have had a pretty good night, after I had eaten my breakfast and was preparing to get ready to go off at 10.00 a.m. I felt something cold running down my leg. Yes, sure thing, it must have opened up again. So I packed plenty of tissues around the knee and more below, so stopping any flow from going down my leg, and bound it all with Microtape. When I arrived, the nurse took me in straightaway and took off all the gear that I had packed around it, keeping some for Mr Mac to inspect. It was some time before he saw me, when he asked me what had occurred. I told him I'd thought it was healing nicely since Wednesday when I'd last seen him, then this morning it had all burst out again. Rubbing his chin (I knew then that some very careful thinking was taking place), he said, 'The swab we took shows it's negative. The blood test is up a little but that is understandable.' As I still have an infection, Mr Mac make my appointment for Wednesday, saying he could do the operation on Thursday. I said, 'I felt this was going to be the outcome. Does that mean I shall have to keep the stitches in for a fortnight and use the CPM?' It was then that Mr Mac mentioned Xmas, continuing in the same tone of voice, 'What are you doing for Xmas?' As I hadn't even thought that far, I just said meekly, 'It's been difficult to arrange, as this has been such a long time getting better.'

The nurse put a fresh dressing on and gave me some more Microtape, which I found to be a godsend for keeping the dressing on.

December 9th

Getting up at 8.10 a.m. I must say I had a pretty good night, with no discharge from the wound.

It's been a very sharp frost and am so glad that the dahlias are indoors for it's now over twenty years that I have kept this *Kidds Climax* variety going: so, like me, if they could talk, they could also write a book on how they have been pushed from pillar to post—so ensuring that all my stories are gospel!

Resting most of the day—well, writing letters, typing and preparing whatever.

I can quite understand how people get addicted to the television because it has certainly got me hooked whilst I am waiting for my health to improve. In the *TV Times*, I look to see what's on, then if there is a programme that I want to watch, I simply cannot wait for the time to come around to turn on. I was eagerly looking forward to watching something at 20.30 hours when the set decided to provide a big flash!!!! Then nothing. Try as I might, I could not get it started, moving the aerial all around!!! Nothing!!!.

As the dressing seemed secure with no discharge, I went to bed leaving it in place.

December 10th

Another new week starting. Up at 7.10 a.m. after a reasonable night. The dressing hardly marked, so was it holding? Outside—another sharp frost, so I walked down to get the weekday paper, well wrapped up. This started the discharge and straightaway when I came back I changed everything—same colour.

A big job I started and completed was defrosting the fridge; also all my laundry delivered, washed and dried and completed before 13.00, among many other chores, all vital ones of everyday life.

Kept the dressing on all day and well into the evening. In fact, changing it was one of the last jobs before I went to bed, there being very little muck on any part of the dressing.

December 11th

With no leaks—I did not have a bad night—I did the same as yesterday, went for the newspaper and then changed the dressing. When I looked, by its appearance it is certainly healing for there has not been any discharge; but it looks angry because of the redness running down both sides, where the stitch marks are.

Lovely day outside, did some chores, then completed approximately thirty Xmas cards. 23.30 hours—the last dressing for the day. It's a bit mucky but hardly anything to write about.

December 12th

Must have had a good night for I have only recorded that after taking off the dressing, it looks as if it's drying up and healing nicely. 7.10—went for a paper and nothing unforeseen has occurred and the wound is holding. Mind you, I don't travel like I would normally do and yet I don't dawdle—just careful with just a nice steady walking pace. This even then to people who know how I move about, with plenty of zip in my step—must make them say, 'Poor old bugger!!!' And yet thinking about this now I've put this in print—do people notice each other like they did in days gone by? (Sorry about this, I digress.)

Completed more Xmas cards rest of morning, also other jobs. This afternoon I have an appointment with Mr Mac.

Saw him just after 15.00 hours and after inspecting the wound and asking me a few questions, he thinks it's apparently healing. He said, 'Now it's healing, we will cancel the bed for tomorrow.'

'That's good,' I said to him quite bluntly, 'but I feel it's going down the same road as before,' pointing to the scab forming, and continuing, 'When it lifted off last time, look at all the anxiety it gave us.'

'No, this looks different this time,' was his reply to this. I also mentioned to him about the swelling directly under my knee on the underside: 'Nothing to worry about. It's probably a cyst. However, we will do a blood test, then make an appointment for next Wednesday.' I said to the nurse after he had gone, 'You feel the heat that's generating from around the knee! And what's the blood test for?' The answer: 'To see if the wound is infected or healing up.' I rest my case. A nice new dressing was applied and an appointment made for 13.45 on December 19th. When I got back home I phoned round to various people to say that I am not going into hospital after all but as I walk round inside the house wearing a pair of shorts and every now and then look at the knee in question, I know it does not seem right when comparing the two because it is a fair size.

December 13th

I did not have a bad night's rest, though the wrapping that I had placed round had come off during the night. But my!! It does ache. Took a couple of PKs straightaway, time—7.10 a.m. Went and picked up paper, leaving the dressing on, did some shopping, all completed before 12.00. Afternoon, I finished some more Xmas cards and opened and read all my post which included all my paperwork for admission to Holly House Hospital today (now cancelled).

I have not changed the dressing all day but just before bedtime I put a fresh one on. It looks good but very red and swollen.

December 14th

Up at 7.10 a.m. Nothing has perforated—so I am going to keep the dressing on and put another dry one over the old one.

Paper, breakfast, read paper and crosswords. I decided to try to do some exercises on the bed. I feel it's important for I have not done anything for some time as we have been waiting for it to heal.

Later on I phoned the television chap who, during the evening, brought a portable one round for me, whilst taking the old one away for replacement parts.

23.45 hours—I changed the dressing which was nice and dry, the swelling about the same, with very little change in its size.

December 15th

I had a disturbance in the night, nothing to do with my operation or anything associated with it. However, it did disturb my sleep at 4.00 a.m. so that I could not go back to sleep afterwards. When I got up at 8.15 a.m. a discharge had started, the same colour as before, and as I was changing the dressings, I considered again for the umpteenth time—why me?!!! Back from shopping, this being Saturday, so I'd had to get my supplies in for the coming week. I then read my correspondence, wrote letters including more accounts to settle, all completed by early afternoon when I started watching the racing!! Then the starter on the portable would not work!

Changed the dressing at 23.30 hours—just a little discharge.

December 16th

Have not had a bad night. I was up at 8.00 a.m. It has discharged a little but nothing much to write home about. I was cheered up later in the afternoon when I had five winners out of six selections!!! No! Hard luck for they were all short-priced favourites after Alan the tele man had come in and repaired the starter!

Later still, I had a phone call from Sue, the retired staff nurse inquiring after my well-being and concerned how I was coping with domestic chores. I told her that the leg is discharging still but not quite so bad and yes, it is still swollen. No, I am not too pleased with it at all.

December 17th

Up at 7.00 a.m. Put a fresh dressing on. After a reasonable night, the wound appears to be the same shape as it was two months ago. Went for paper.

Later on took a bottle of my single malt whisky round to one of my neighbours where we wished each other a very happy Xmas—with a few glasses.

11.45 hours. The wound looked fairly clean when I changed the final dressing for the day.

December 18th

I had a lie-in this morning for it was 7.25 a.m., before I got up, so decided to leave dressing on until later. Went for paper.

As the shop was not open, the papers had been left outside by the deliveryman, so everyone was helping themselves to their favourite daily. Am pretty sure as I have now lived down here in Loughton for a few years those payments would be made when staff turned up. How do I know that, you might ask? I am confident that the regular customers coming through those doors would feel guilty if they had not paid their dues—I know you cannot judge a person as quick as that, yet I like to think that my judgment would be ninety per cent correct.

When I came back I had to change my dressing—and what a mess! I decided to try somehow to improve this, for when I had cleaned it all up with the antiseptic provided, the little tiny hole was now clearly visible and went down some way into the depths. So I packed more tissues around the final part so if and when the oozing started then this would act as a good absorbent. Did not do much for the rest of the day—just rested up.

Before I went to bed at approximately 23.30 hours, I took off all the old dressings and packing and replaced it with a new gauze dressing, then the dressing and finally several tissues as the final covering, then a towel wrapped round the whole lot. Then with the bath towel laid across the bed I felt well prepared for any emergency.

December 19th

I have to see Mr Mac today at 13.45 and though I have not had a bad night, as I have recorded, there is still a lot of concern over the future of my knee, especially after my seeing it this morning with all the filthy stuff that has been discharging during the night. After tidying it all up and putting on a fresh dressing. I went for the paper where I offered to pay for the newspaper from the day before. 'No, you don't want to do that. The management knew that the chap in charge was having a day off. That's their bad luck!!!'

My appointment was for 13.45 hours, but it was some time before he was able to see me. When he did, the Outpatients' nurse had uncovered and tidied up the wound for him to inspect. The wound was still discharging in front of him. 'That's it. Come in tomorrow for an operation, give it a good wash out and we'll get it sorted,' Mr Mac said and did I note a hint of despair in his voice? I shook his hand and reminded him that— I think he has done his best for me with eighty-four tablets, several swabs and blood tests.

Back home—more phone calls to say that I have got to go into Holly House Hospital after all and should have it all washed out to find out where the infection has originated from. Keep your fingers crossed for me—to most of them.

Final dressings at 23.45 hours. I replaced the old dressing with a new one and made it all secure for the night with a final good lot of packing around the whole lot.

December 20th

I was up at 6.45 a.m. Straightaway I put a fresh dressing on, for there had been a fair bit of discharge below the knee. I cleaned this all up with tissues, then paper and delivered Xmas cards. As I am nil by mouth after 8.00 a.m. I make sure I have a decent breakfast which includes two poached eggs on toast. Completed all my duties, which was quite a handful if I was to article them off. It would take several pages but this space is valuable for my next visit and final one, I thought, to Holly House Hospital.

The Accounts lady welcomed me and took me to Room 135 where I told her that the claim number on my file would be the same as before, as I had been in touch with the insurance company. The young lady very politely, on the phone had told me, 'We understand the situation and realise that it has to be done and hope all goes well.'

I was quickly asked by the staff nurse taking my notes, when was the last time I had taken any food. 'About 7.30 a.m. and nothing since.' 'Good,' was her reply.

Mr Mac came round at 13.30, asked me if there were any questions I wanted to ask him. 'No,' I said, shaking his hand, wishing him the best of luck. I then signed up to say I authorised him to cut me up again. He then marked up the leg to be operated on. There did not appear to be any hold-ups for my position on his list of operations. For making enquiries now and again, seemingly everything was going according to schedule or possibly the clock on the wall was playing tricks with my vision. Pretty sure the time—17.00 hours—Mr Dodd and the theatre staff soon did the necessary and back in the ward at 20.30 hours.

I am not sure if I read the situation correctly but it would not have been unusual for I came to witness this many times—the nurses on duty were worried that their charge had been gone a long time. When I had sufficiently recovered I was offered something to eat and drink. I refused as I couldn't eat a thing.

23.30—I had an injection, sleeping and painkillers.

December 21st

I had a good night. The night nurse called in at 6.00 a.m. to give me an injection of antibiotics in the bottom and arm.

After eating my breakfast cereals, BB and two pieces of toast I got out of bed, went to the toilet, washed and shaved and found that the huge bandage that had been wrapped round was not too much of an obstacle despite what it looked like, for it appeared to be very cumbersome!!!! I would just have to chance what it looked like.

During the morning—another injection—bottom and arm.

12.20 hours—lunch arrives, ate the lot with all the Mrs Moppses arriving to bring me an Xmas tree. After my first meeting with the youngest M/s Mopp, I said, 'Whew, what a Super Girl!' Xmas cards and a balloon with get well wishes on it—for all like me knew there was no going home for Xmas and, I had not even considered this, but perhaps the New Year too. Then of course, when I am thinking along those lines, my holiday in New Zealand might also be affected.

By 13.15 hours I started feeling dozy and also am drinking a fair drop of water, perhaps because of the injections and antibiotics. As well as this I have logged that I have heartburn and pains across the chest, but when my observations are made, blood pressure, pulse and temperature are all good.

At 8.20 hours dinner is served. I had ordered chicken, peas, mash and, for dessert, apple pie and custard. A cuppa arrives about twenty minutes later. I had consumed all this fine fare and had just picked up the newspaper again when Mr Mac called in, asking me how I was feeling, telling me that he had cut it open, going down to where it had started discharging; everything had been cleaned and given a good wash out. He continued, 'We'll have to wait and see. The source might well be in the bone itself! If so, we will have to start afresh.' I looked at him in amazement and felt really deflated. He knew how I was feeling, for I was saying nothing for once. He then rubbed more salt into the now rapidly expanding wounds around my body, by further confirmation! Yes—new knee replacements, as the infection could well be in that area. I asked him, 'Am I an unusual case?'

'Yes, you are about one per cent.'

I didn't read the paper, as there were other things on my

mind, particularly Mr Mac's last remark that I was one per cent, for this had really knocked me for six. As soon as he had passed on this information I thought straightaway how I believed that, one day, one per cent would catch up with me. I'd been in the building trade, motor cycling, and in many activities where at times high risk was the name of the game, so I could not grumble! I have lived a long life and avoided that one per cent for more years now than I can remember. Back to reality, I picked up the phone, letting those that want to know my latest misfortunes.

To cheer me up my Xmas and Get Well cards are now going up round the room and, as it is a tiny room, most everyone who comes in finds it difficult to manoeuvre around other pieces of furniture. But who am I to complain? After all, the staff seem to cope excellently with these handicaps—whatever annoyances arise, they just seem to be breezed away.

December 22nd

I have had a pretty good night though I must have done some wriggling for the drain came out during the night and was now dripping onto the floor carpet. The same as my other operations, there is a one-pound jam jar for the liquid to drain into—and my word it is some dreadful-looking stuff. It is all part of the cleansing of the blood, which makes sure that only pure blood circulates.

Night nurses give me my injections and tablets. Other times for these during the day are 12.00 and 18.00 hours.

Mr Mac came round at about 14.00 hours and leaves instructions for the drain pipe to be removed as well as taking off the large crepe bandage and replacing it with a smaller one. After this duty was completed I went to the toilet and found that a thoughtful nurse had added an attachment to raise the seat and now, with the big bandage removed, this indeed was like sitting in the Ritz!!! (Well, it's in London somewhere and I'm not likely to visit.) I did just have one problem today and that was associated with my 12.00 hours injection. There was nobody in the nursing department who had sufficient knowledge to stick this in the two-way plug attached to the back of my hand. There was only a delay of ten minutes while a senior staff had to be relocated to my room for this important part of my recovery. The same thing occurred later on. After this third operation, I now realise that pills and medicines will arrive, but very seldom on time. This should not be to the detriment of anyone! This does not have any after-effects in any shape or form; as I have mentioned before, it's all about workload and staffing levels.

December 23rd

6.20 a.m. The night nurse has given me my jabs and you realise how it is important to inject the antibiotics very slowly into the back of the hand via a Vac-Flo. This took a good five minutes to empty for it was a mixture of two ingredients, both liquids totalling several milligrams each. I was told that injecting slowly is the correct method. I am told: 'There should not be any after-effects now,' followed by a look of reassurance. Who am I to disagree? I thought this might be the last time I think about after-effects but it was not to be.

Soon after breakfast, I had asked the day nurse on duty for the mattress to be changed if possible, as it was playing hell with me and my need to lie on my side trying to sleep. I did not realise how much I nag but as other staff joined in the search for the comfort of yours truly, it made me feel quite important. One was eventually found, it was placed on the bed for my approval—very good! Then a monkey pole was soon found as the one currently attached did not suit me or the bed either.

12.30 hours—for about half an hour, the Salvation Army turned up outside the main entrance doors and played some nice melodies. It appeared that one of their officers was an incumbent in a room at the front of the hospital—yes, of course I went to the window to see them perform together with several others who were not involved with duties. I am sure the gentleman concerned much appreciated this very nice Xmas gesture.

The resident doctor came along later to give me my injection. I suppose there was a reason for this. I certainly know that there was a bigger time gap than when I had received the last lot, same arm, same liquids, almost the same time. I told him that my arm was aching a little, but put it down to the blood pressure—very seldom the same reading! High blood pressure?

December 24th

The sister is on the ball at 6.00 a.m. and looked at my arm, saying she was not very happy with its condition as it was swollen.

After breakfast, I was out reading the paper whilst the nurses were changing the sheets, asking them—as there is a lot of activity—what was going on? The senior staff says that they are closing down parts of this wing and moving everyone who is staying over for Xmas into Cedar Ward and those that are able are going home. By this time a sister on duty had arrived, looked at my arm and within a short time, the resident doctor had arrived and changed the two-way plug into my other arm. For it appeared that difficulty to get into the vein had been a problem with the one used originally.

After lunch at about 13.00 hours, Mr Mac arrived, had a look at his work; with just a little discharge, he seemed happy. A fresh dressing was put on as soon as he left, but no mention of the CPM machine which I thought might be applied by this time. I do realise that it is important for it to heal, so as this was only the fourth day following the operation I mustn't be in too big a hurry to get back to doing my exercises. It was not long before it was my turn to be moved. Back into Room 151 which was a much bigger room with a nice view onto where the builders were putting a new tiled roof on the physio department.

It was fortunate that my cousin and his wife had arrived, so they were able to give the nurses a hand with my now considerable collection of Xmas, Get Well cards, flowers, etc. to my new address in 151 Cedar Ward (an address that I was not to know I was going to get used to). Senior sister tells me that after all the changing about has quietened down, I am to have my antibiotics in tablet form and not by injection any more.

There has been a delay about having my tablets, as the resident doctor has to sign the form permitting this changeover from injection to tablet. This was quickly sorted out and I was once again sleeping with an untroubled mind. At 22.00 hours I have to take my last tablets for the day, observations are taken and it's found that I am running a temperature (little did I know what was in store for me next day).

Xmas Day, December 25th

Am off to a bad start—I have taken a tablet at 6.15 hours. This is to do with keeping at bay the infection that I'd had previously. During the night at 1.00 a.m. I had asked the night sister to let me have a sleeping tablet because I could not sleep.

This was in addition to the one I had taken before I went to sleep. At 7.00 a.m. the indigestion started. I said that I had taken the earlier ones on an empty stomach. I was given some Gaviscon and also suggestions that I do some walking to move the wind. But my tummy pains were not better, in fact worse, because the staff on duty decided to call the resident doctor who brought the ECG machine with him. I was then wired up, telling him that I had yesterday undergone the change from the arm to tablet form with the antibiotics plus the tablets taken this morning. He left me saying he would phone Dr Dodd to see if he would call in. Within twenty minutes, Mr Mac had arrived. Telling him how the stomach was not all that happy, I welcomed him with a couple of burps—which I am sure afterwards he suspected I did on purpose. I told him about what I had told the other doctor. He then said, 'It must be the Voltarol tablets. Stop taking them and then we will see how it goes.' He said to the sister, 'We'll try him on Codydramol and see how that helps him.' By this time the Xmas lunch had arrived and my word it did look nice with a couple of parsnips done just as I like them for Xmas. Yet I hardly ate a thing!!!! I know for certain that this is the only Xmas meal that I have never enjoyed, not even the Xmas pudding and cream specially purchased for the dozen or so patients in the whole building to partake of, for this very special day.

13.30 hours, I have to take another tablet, the same sort as before but to be changed later to one called Flucloxacillin One of the senior sisters turned up, reminding me that this was not the first time I had had digestive troubles. 'You are quite right,' I replied, 'but I can't recall it being as bad as this.' Had I been walking?' 'Yes.' I have been out several times, sometimes just moving around the bed.

I suppose it would have been about half an hour later that I decided to start doing exercises, some on the bed, just moving my feet and stretching the muscles with the quads contractions that I know are beneficial to me. I then noticed some blood oozing through the dressing, so called the staff on duty who removed the old one to find that it was weeping. A better dressing was applied; it was now about mid-afternoon on Xmas Day when I would be normally preparing to put my feet up, feeling contented. Everything seemed to be holding, there was just the faintest of weeping coming through, but the staff came back to say she would put another dressing on over the existing one which would then help the situation. Then panic!!! From this small hole it did not seem possible that I was witness to what was occurring in front of my eyes. She said, 'Press the button, Perc,' for the blood would not stop. It was coming out in a fine spray through her hands, no matter how hard she pressed on the area. Two other nurses arrived very quickly including the senior sister, who immediately said, 'Get the doctor down here quick and phone Mr Mac as well.' A tourniquet was then placed tightly around the area but the blood continued to flow. By this time Mr Mac had phoned in to say, 'Get his leg up in the air,' which the resident doctor was now in the throes of doing. It was fortunate that I had got used to the monkey pole for I was able to help the nursing staff gathered round my bed. If my memory serves me correctly it was a South African doctor who was on duty at the time and I was gently and carefully manoeuvred to a position whereby my head was tucked into my chest and my leg was supported by pillows on the end of the bed. However ridiculous I looked, I knew it was important that I kept in this position for some considerable time, several hours, which is what Mr Mac had suggested. The doctor stayed around to see if all was well, so I was left to console myself in this strange position that I had never expected to be in—hardly able to breathe, with the leg at an angle. I even refused the Xmas cake which had arrived during the mêlée. However, when the dust had settled I was still presented with a piece later on in Room 151. None of us had expected this to happen, for there had been no warning; it had come about only when I started doing those exercises on the bed. I must admit that the situation was always under control and those involved dealt with the situation with extreme professionalism. Reviewing the situation I now found myself in, all I could watch was the wall clock on the right side, hanging on the wall above the built-in wardrobe. I kept glancing at it every few seconds, so you can rest assured that these few hours were going to be the longest that I have ever spent; I was only able to move my head to and fro, and let my right leg have an occasional wriggle

It was about 19.30 hours when the staff nurse came in to check my leg and found that it was still weeping blood, so a fresh dressing was placed on the wound. I realised that I could not move until it was safe to warrant it. Earlier in the day when Mr Mac had called when I had my gastric problems, he said that as the Voltarol tablets could be causing all the concern I was to stop taking them for the time being. When the trolley came along with the pills, medicines and tablets, I was given a couple of antibiotics together with a glass of milk and a few biscuits. I remember that I hoped and prayed that I would never ever have another Xmas Day like today has been.

December 26th

I have had a shocking night, for I have had to keep my head cranked up, supported by pillows, still with my legs on the incline. The night nurse has been in several times to readjust the pillows for me.

I don't recall any staff about until about 8.30 a.m. Am sure nobody has rung a buzzer so most everyone is happy with what Santa so far has brought them for Christmas. Am pretty sure that I must have disturbed a lot of the room's patients with my performance the latter part of yesterday. All my observations have been completed. I have some Gaviscon before my breakfast which was only cereals, then the usual pills plus one I am now taking called Augmentin. During the day I have Gaviscon for the gastric troubles, antibiotics to keep clearing the blood, and in between I'm drinking and eating fruit.

Mr Mac called in at 16.30 hours to see how I was, for I had been lying in a normal way, with my legs and head in respectable positions. He told me that I was just to potter about—no bending of the leg, keep it quiet. West Ham had won today 4-0 against Derby County.

At 22.30 hours the sister in charge brought me in a cup of hot chocolate together with pills and a few biscuits.

December 27th

3.00 a.m. I felt something cold in bed! Blood!!!! I rang the buzzer for the sister who came to investigate what had occurred this time. Seeing the blood, this was one sister who, like the others, just took this in her stride. She quickly took off the dressing to find it had stopped but the bed was in a pretty pickle for it had gone right through the sheets and to the mattress below. She put a tight crepe bandage round the offending object, then all the bedlinen had to be changed. Fortunately very little had got onto my shorts, which I found, after my first visit, were the best things to wear in bed; nevertheless as soon as I went to the toilet I made a change.

Breakfast arrived with what I had ordered the night before— I ate two poached eggs on two pieces of toast with baked beans, eating the lot, also taking my tablets with this meal. I had not realised how large a bandage the sister had put on, but if it was doing its job—so well and good. This is the day I also have a change of antibiotics. During the day not only do I meet several boarders but also have several visitors myself, telling them and making them laugh about my Xmas Day exploits and misdemeanours. One asked surely not all on Xmas Day? 'On my life,' I replied. Then at 15.45 hours, having enjoyed my lunch earlier, a piece of Xmas cake arrived, not one but two pieces. I was not to do any walking, only potter, like Mr Mac said on his last visit—so this is what I was doing. I'm sure my Xmas cake approves.

The Flucloxacillin, together with my usual tablets, must be beneficial to my getting back on the right road again.

December 28th

Sister round early with the trolley at 6.00 a.m. Have also had all my observations done. By 8.30 a.m. I have had my early morning cuppa, my breakfast, tablets, wash, shave, tidy-up. My pyjama top has been washed and dried during the night so all nice and clean for the new day. I am told the dressing has to stay on all day.

12.00 hours—scampi, chips and peas—ate the lot including the dessert of fruit and ice cream. I had several visitors during the day and in between company I decided to have a walk along to the ward where I had come from. I had reached the end and was looking into a room, hearing someone cough. I said, 'Is anyone in there and if so would you like a visitor?'

'By all means, come in,' the reply came. I made myself known to him and he to me. After we had a chat about the weather outside which was extremely windy and blowing a gale, he told me something that I thought most unusual and that was he had been coming here for six and a half years for treatment to improve his well-being and I was the first one in all that time who had ever made himself known to him. At first I could not believe this was the case, and he could see that I was taken aback by this remark!!! Then quickly regaining control of my grey matter, I said, 'Well, if you say so, then it must be so. I dare say you have been asleep when people like myself have passed by and they have called out.'

'No, you are a first, I can assure you. All I hear is walking and exercising, that's all.' I stopped for a good half an hour and by that time, found that we both knew various associates around the district, especially when I told him that I had been nearly forty years in the building trade and had worked in several streets in the area he came from. Of course talking to him and regaling him with some of my trade stories made him forget his problems. Then when it came to my local church, High Beech, he told me that it was a place that he liked to visit and just sit on one of the seats to become involved with the peace, calmness and serenity of the churchyard and the surrounding forest. I told him that I do not go into the church much for services but I did help to keep tidy part of the churchyard —where my family were laid to rest. I do know that, after shaking his hand, wishing him well, passing on a fair bit of information about High Beech that he had not heard during his time around the district, and a few other things, I had made him laugh on several occasions and I left him with a contented mind!!! Passing, one of the staff nurses asked me where I had been and who I had visited, for it was now getting to be quite common knowledge that Percy went visiting. I don't mind telling you that it made my day when I had been told I was a first!!!!

I had enjoyed the roast lamb cutlets, potatoes, cauliflower, carrots and apple pie and custard for my dinner and also had had another piece of Xmas cake earlier. I was eating and felt much better as the day progressed.

I had taken sleeping tablets only a short time before lights out, confident that I was going to have a good night.

December 29th

Pretty good night, early morning cuppa at 7.20 a.m. All observations taken and all right. Breakfast at 8.00 a.m. With this I am now taking my tablets which I have been counting—as it is fifteen a day, I have logged—'I must get better after all this lot!'

Wash, shave, back washed, then the dressing was changed. It doesn't look too bad, there is a slight weeping of blood coming from the same place as before. I think this must be a weak spot, so no doubt it will take a fair time to close and heal.

The staff nurse has completed the new dressing and taped it all up securely, when I told her of the various methods different nurses have with dressings, and that hers was one that was very different from the rest. I didn't half get a mouthful, and was glad when she said, 'It looks all right to me,' leaving me to dwell on the state of affairs below the dressing. I am sure in retrospect it makes no difference for it's the end result that counts. Had several more visitors bringing cards for me. I must have something like sixty now. During the afternoon I watched horse racing with the friend who lives round the corner who had come along too.

A chap who has been a patient here was going home today so we both saw him off along the corridor wishing him well.

I had the dressing changed after dinner as it was oozing through again.

Sleeping tablet just before lights out.

December 30th

Have had a pretty good night. I had some early pills soon after the trolley came round at 6.45 a.m. but I always tell the sister in charge that I prefer to take them with food, for I always maintain that my tummy problems were caused by the tablets I had taken on an empty stomach!!! This did not seem to interfere with the book of knowledge (my chart book) which is always registered as duty performed!

After all my dailies have been undertaken and I am sitting reading the newspaper one of the sisters comes along and wants to have a look at the wound, removing the dressing to find that it is still weeping blood, but she says, 'It's looking good.' The large bandage is replaced with a smaller one which is only covering the thigh part of the operation. There are quite a few new patients who have had knee and hip surgery so decided to pop round and have a chat with them. Lawrence, the chap in Room 149, had had a hip operation like I had seven years ago but his one has a different type of fixing and I am pleased to say he is making tremendous progress. Yes, of course, we had met several times whilst walking together with another chap who was in Room 148 called Eric. When I started talking to him, it soon became apparent to us all that cricket was at the forefront of our thoughts, especially as the Tour Groups for New Zealand are preparing for travel and of course he was mightily interested when I told him that I was going with the England party to see the three test matches and was hoping and praying that my knee was going to be healed and ready for action within the next month or two. He was a local chap, very much involved with local cricket who not only played against a lot of the teams I had played against but also, as he was now in the twilight of his career, had taken up umpiring and had almost completed his final exams for doing this thankless job. He told me that he had waited two years for this hip operation so was not looking forward to the next six weeks. Of course I told him about the banner, which he had seen, through the years—the High Beech logo with Essex on—wondering who it belonged to. As I said at the time, 'I plead guilty.' He was also a keen supporter of the West Ham FC so whenever they or my team Spurs were playing a game, there was always friendly rivalry. As there were also other patients who favoured other football teams, so the general topics were football and cricket.

As you realise, this visiting had occupied most of the morning, so it was fortunate when midday arrived that I only had to walk across the corridor to 151.

An assortment of cream crackers were awaiting me together with a selection of cheeses, all presented on various varieties of lettuce leaves.

More exercises in the afternoon (walking) as well as visiting the top floor, which was still quiet for the New Year was just around the corner and, judging by the Holly House Hospital grapevine, the coming week was going to be a busy one.

Dinner—one of my favourites—scampi, peas, fish fingers with apple crumble and custard. 22.45—painkillers and sleeping tablets, lights out 23.00 hours.

December 31st

The last day of the old year and what a lot of New Year resolutions I have to remember for later on.

All the observations completed before 7.00 a.m. The early morning cuppa arrived at 7.30 a.m. and outside it was what it should always be on the last day, a very sharp frost and very cold, judging by the staff as they came on duty—reminding me that what a nice warm room I had with many comforts to be getting along with. One of the staff pointed this out, and I offered the same reply as usual and that was: 'I would willingly give up all these luxuries for my health and strength back so that I could wander in the forest, kicking and jumping like a young gazelle.' I should be so lucky.

By 9.30 I had completed breakfast, all my other duties, and had read part of Monday's paper; I'd also had my feet washed and cleaned, and white stockings put on. This task was more difficult than you can imagine, for not many of the nursing staff got it right first time. In fact, two nurses did it differently when on duty, yet had been trained by the same person at the London Hospital. What mattered most was that the completed pair stayed in the right place with no sign of a big toe peeping through and in my case I cannot recall this ever occurring. The staff nurse looking after me today has decided not to interfere with the dressing. I told her it had been on for a long time, since late the previous evening. I said, 'I think it should be changed.' Of course my day's affairs had been discussed at the early changeover, which nobody informs you of. All have their little pieces of paper with the patients' needs for the day carefully placed in order of importance, given to them as they are allocated their tasks for their shift.

I had a walk up to the second floor via the lift, had a steady wander along the wing, where there is now a very thriving cosmetic service which patients can receive at a reasonable cost, I am told. All the staff are the same here as elsewhere, very friendly and helpful. Have a chat with the two lads about football on the way back.

Lunch at 12.00 hours: cream crackers, various cheeses with a tomato, dessert rice pudding and jam.

Nobody can view any racing (horses) for all has been called off owing to ice and frost.

A chap much senior to me, in Room 144 has had to go

for an ultrasound scan, so when he came back, as he kept pressing his bell, I called in to have a chat with him. As I told him I had not been a football secretary for twenty-five years for nothing, as players' problems were always top of the list. I might have given wrong advice sometimes, but I always said how often do the experts get it right?—and they are paid thousands. This time unfortunately, of all his friends, there is no one who can take charge of his insurance and this indeed is a sorry state for sums and the like are well down on my list for cheering a person up with good advice to make sure they will have a contented mind when I leave.

His doctor came to see him just before the afternoon tea break—I have recorded that he had a voice like our old vicar, Reverend Walter Jones, our priest before, during and after the Second World War.

Mr Mac called in at 15.30 hours. The dressing was removed to find it had expressed very little discharge. Then, with the nurse making notes of his orders, he tells me that as the stitches have been in nearly fourteen days come Wednesday: 'They can come out, then see how it feels. You can then go home.'

After he had gone, I think, if he wants me to go home, I am going to find it mighty difficult to bend my knee for I have not attempted to do any CPM exercises as the orders have always been, 'We must let it heal, then the bending can come later.' I must also make sure which day I am going home this time, for I did not want to surprise either myself or my relatives and friends about a coming-home day. Another dressing had been put in place with Microtape, seems good all round. Dinner at 18.30 hours—bourguignon, mushrooms, etc., etc., dessert creamed rice with apple crumble. The night shift had taken over round about 21.00 hours and as it appears that there are not many patients to look after, the order came round that there would be some non-alcoholic bubbly arriving. Well you never know there might be something stronger.

New Year's Eve

The dressing was to stop on and at 22.00 hours my pills arrived together with my sleeping tablets. Lights out at 23.00 hours!!! I was told early the next morning that I had been asleep when the bubbly came round so I was not to be disturbed. I asked the sister who gave me this information, 'When did the fireworks start, because I certainly heard them?' 'Midnight,' came the reply—I rest my case. This I do remember; there certainly was a lot of nattering going on out in the corridor for I have obviously recorded this the next day when I was reading through my notes.

January 1st 2001

Confirming what I overheard in the corridor this morning I said to the night sister that she must have opened and closed my door pretty quickly. In any case everybody was wishing each other all the very best for the New Year and this continued right through the day. By 8.45 a.m. all my dailies had been completed, with the breakfast understandably a bit later than usual. By 9.30 the linen had been changed. I asked the staff in charge about the dressing. 'Don't you think it ought to come off being the first day of the New Year?' I suggested to her. 'No,' came the reply, 'it is staying on all day.'

By 10.30 a.m. no papers were forthcoming. After wishing Lawrence, Eric and a few others the New Year greetings, as they did not have any newspapers either, I offered to sort the problem out. I asked one of our reliables, the senior Mrs Mopp, the one who when I first made her acquaintance I named Mrs

SP (shot putter) if she would pop across the road and get some newspapers for us. 'No problem,' and the task was quickly undertaken and everyone had their selection. None of us had the same one—all different. After a good read, I went for another walk, wishing more patients and staff New Year good wishes.

12.20 hours, my lunch arrives. I am realising that only non-fatty foods are going to be the priority, now that home day is arriving, so just a cream crackers assortment, also cheeses, a tomato sliced up and a small bunch of grapes, rice pudding and jam and of course little packets of butter (spread very thinly). Then several phone calls incoming and outgoing.

As there was not a lot on the box and the Sky television needed some repairs done to it, it looked like it was going to be a bleak afternoon. This indeed was the case, several football matches off, and all of the racing except for one all-weather track, all due to the hard frost in most parts of the UK.

We have another staff sister in charge this afternoon. Whilst talking to her, she tells me she is a councillor, but am not clear with what business she might be connected!!!! A counsellor in the medical profession, or a local councillor?!! I am only sorry that I failed to make further inquiries. Through to dinner, the first one in the New Year, served up on the dot. I had ordered a lamp chop, magic. Together with mint sauce, new potatoes, Brussels, carrots, and then apple pie and custard. Had my usual walk to keep exercising. That was most important, I knew. All the physio girls made sure that I did not forget this either.

It was between those hours after dinner and before late drinks at 21.00 hours that I asked the sister in charge if she should look at the dressing. 'I will later'—her reply. I told her that nobody had looked at it now since it was last changed at about 16.00 hours yesterday and by the time Mr Mac calls it might well have been on for two whole days. 'Leave it with me, Percy.' I was concerned as if it was still discharging slightly, there was no way he was going to authorise removing all those stitches—about forty-two I have counted—before I went home. Sure thing, 21.00 hours, sister came round, took off the old dressing: 'Magic, dry as a bone. There you are, Percy, nothing to worry about.' Then fixing a light dressing on, I felt there was good progress at last. I am going to sleep well tonight after taking my sleepers. With the first day out of the way, was I going to have all the good health that so many people had been wishing me?

January 2nd

I had a good night—peace of mind at last as the healing has set in—for what I thought was permanently.

6.40 a.m.—all the observations completed, the early morning cuppa girl says, 'It's freezing outside with ice—a nasty morning to come into work.'

Breakfast 8.30 a.m. Had some extra toast this morning with my poached eggs, completed with marmalade.

Staff nurse is giving me extras this morning for not only feet are washed, also legs—stockings are changed and the dirty ones rinsed out. I told her not to do that because it gives me something to do. Then a walk to see how Lawrence and Eric, my two closest neighbours are getting on. It's remarkable really, for Eric, the more senior one of our trio is going great guns and it will not be long before he is discharged. Mind you, all due respect to him, but both Lawrence and me are somewhat rounder than him, and we're both a lot taller. All of us have had our operations done by Mr Mac, who must be well pleased with their progress. The morning soon went, all the patients who were able to move about were back in their rooms, when

12.00 hours and the lunch trolley arrived. Yesterday I had enjoyed the pickled onion that came along with the assorted cream crackers and cheeses, so today I had the same plus a tomato, with apple crumble as a dessert with custard. Early afternoon, I went for a walk along the corridor, and was talking to Marjorie, a coloured lady who was having a replacement hip problem sorted out when Mr Mac came in. After he had had a chat with her, he asked me how I was getting on. 'Fine,' I replied. He went on: 'You can have your stitches out tomorrow, then you can go home.' Thanking him I said, 'Will it be all right if I go home next day—Friday, as I have to arrange several things?'

'Yes, okay,' was his reply with a nod of his head.

Now I had to start my round of telephone calls to let different people know that I was coming home on Friday January 4th and that was sure. Phoning the retired sister Sue, I said that all seemed under control and that the stitches would be out tomorrow.

18.00 hours dinner arrived and as it was a full house and I was in the mood to tuck in I ate everything, roast chicken, stuffing, roast and new potatoes, Brussels, peas, cabbage, rice pudding and an apple that my friend, the postie Tony had brought along.

I had a last walk at 19.00 hours. Lawrence invited me in to watch the football with him, for the person in charge of household duties had pulled out the stops to get the Sky telly put right. I told him that I would rather not as I had some more calls to make and I had to make up the diary!!!! I am sure I did not say anything to him about those notes I was keeping. At 22.30 hours—more pills plus my sleeping tablets. I asked the sister in charge about using the CPM machine. 'We'll see what Mr Mac says. Shortly after this she brought back a message to say, 'Yes, when the dressing and stitches are removed tomorrow. We'll put a lighter dressing on for you though for through the night.'

The football had been a very competitive game with Man UTD (3) Newcastle (1).

January 3rd

6.15 a.m. Did not have a bad night, all observations completed by 6.40 a.m. Early morning cuppa. 7.30 a.m. after breakfast with all regular jobs safely out of the way, I let the staff nurse complete the tasks with a backwash. I was not quite in a position to do this job for myself, as I still had all those stitches to contend with; if I had showered there could have been a slight misfortune which could set me back a bit with my being discharged tomorrow. 10.00 hours: the staff nurse came in together with two agency nurses who were going to watch her take out the metal stitches, then the lower part was sealed with a solution which I am told would not only keep it clean but also has healing purposes as well.

Have jotted down in my diary in brackets: POOR OLD WRITING DESK, SIDE OF GOOD AND BAD LEG. You might wonder what this refers to. As I was lying on the bed, part of both legs formed a splendid easel for my notes that I kept whilst writing on the adjustable wheelie table; it slides over the bed in high or lower positions, its purpose for food and drinks obviously but also useful for other activities.

From her attitude, for one nurse I was confident that it was her first time to see stitches removed and of course I twigged this straightaway as well as the staff—a couple of times, I made as if I was suffering a lot of pain so this particular nurse turned quite a strange colour, while the staff said, 'Sorry, Perc, did I hurt you?' The final one out—she then remarked, 'Wound looks pretty good considering it's been opened three times.' The physiotherapist come in to say that I must not go on CPM as the flesh is too tender so it will have to be done manually.

I said, 'I guessed as much.' I don't mind telling you I was really getting concerned for it was ages since I had got that machine round to ninety-five degrees. Physio says, 'Come on, Percy, we have a lot to do.' So bed, side of bed—this for the rest of the morning together with walks along the corridor.

Lunch at 12.00 hours, change of meal today, for ham and eggs were on the menu together with chips, then ice cream with wafer biscuits, apple. Those meals by the way, would always be followed by a cuppa or whatever you required.

13.10 hours I am walking with the physio for the first time to challenge the staircase, of course with my crutches supporting me. I was knackered when I got back to my room!!!! And have underlined in my diary 'KNEE IS A SIZE.' Half as big again as the other knee! I splutter, 'ONE PER CENT!!!! TIME AND PATIENCE,' for my ears only. It takes time to calm down for it has generated a lot of heat during the twenty minutes I have been away.

The new shift takes over at 14.15 hours and as the corridor is busy, have to make sure not too much traffic is about when I go for walkies. Mr Mac today has completed *three* hip operations. During the afternoon, Lawrence's wife came along with her camera, so we all had our photos taken with several of the nurses and staff on duty. I was going up to get myself weighed but as the nurse who could read the machine correctly was not available I had to forget about this.

19.00 hours I made a couple more phone calls as the people were still at work whom I'd wanted to ring earlier. Bad news from Tony, the postie, his brother, Jack had just passed away. I asked him to pass on my condolences.

Mr Mac came round during this period just before late drinks, had a good look at it and said, 'It looks fine.' We both spoke about the machine and how backward I had become in bending the knee, as it was such a long time since I used the CPM. He said, 'If you continue to have trouble with it, in about two months time, I will put you on a manipulating machine after sending you to sleep, then this machine will automatically put it right.' I said, 'My, it does sound painful, I hope it does not come to that.'

January 4th

Have arranged to be home at about 12.30 p.m.

I had something to occupy my mind for most of this time after the early morning cuppa had arrived—saying cheerio to several patients, also the staff who were on duty—my, how well they had looked after me, especially two of the staff who were on duty at Xmas who still do have a laugh at the position I had found myself in on Xmas night. Packing all completed, I had phoned my own Mrs Mopp who would be at home when I arrived and I knew a nice cuppa would not be long in coming forward.

Everything went to plan—taxi, etc., etc. In the afternoon I did plenty of exercises, for I was determined to get the leg bending like the other one, so onto the table—my, this dear old kitchen table could tell a few tales. Its history started towards the end of the nineteenth century and without a word of a lie it has been in action ever since. It had been repaired in 1959; then there was no actual repair work done, only because the pine top had begun to shred splinters Tony Saxon, the carpenter, took pity on dear old Mum and planed the whole surface—thereafter, you can imagine that when it was used it was a case of 'Careful, mind you don't damage it.' I dare say when it was made originally, it would only have cost pence, but it was not how much the thing cost, it was the amount of pleasure it had brought into the household down the hundred-odd years since its birth. Am working on its uses—at fifty I have stopped counting. I had completed my exercises for the time being and was resting up, looking at the knee in question and realising that it isn't half a size. I know I have been told it has been cut about so much internally so I suppose I shall have to go along with it.

A few phone calls and a couple of letters completed the rest of the day, with me taking things steady.

January 5th, 6th, 7th

Over the weekend and Monday, the usual household duties and, in any case, I did not do much, only kept persevering with the exercises—also had a few visitors.

January 8th

Continued with bed, table, settee, weights and ice pack and all important medicines. Have had lots of interest shown in the forthcoming publication of my book *Breakout at Sixty-five* and I tell each person that it is a good read and by no means a rubbishy one. It also includes twelve illustrations.

January 9th

I have marked up a busy day in my diary, not so far as it concerned the healing of my wound but because of other equally important everyday operations: bus to Walthamstow—main reason to purchase a diary to keep my notes in and which I am now writing in back home. Sharp out (typewriter), three letters, envelopes, typed addresses. Then other visitors in the afternoon, then exercises every hour after this. Phone call during the evening—Alan, the telly man is going to bring back my own repaired set again, now he knows I am back home.

The knee is still swollen and, to my way of thinking, there does not appear to be any change. It's still hot as well.

January 10th

Have not mentioned the weather as it has been some time since I saw it for real. This morning, when I went to get my paper, it was pretty dull and overcast. Forecast is for a bright day. Posted all my letters.

As it was going to be nice later, decided to do some washing, so put nine pieces out on the line. Alan, with the repaired television, arrives at 12.00 hours, asking me how the little portable set had behaved. I told him, yes it had been okay but I missed the teletext I usually enjoy on my own set. I asked him if he would like to try a piece of my Victoria sponge. After tasting, eating and obviously enjoying it and sampling another slice, he said, 'You didn't make this, Perc, did you? It's jolly good.'

I have marked down at the end of the day, that I am sure my knee is responding to all my exercises. What a difference a day makes!!! Must be in the mind.

I have now been home for seven days, so I am now almost back in the old routine, collecting the newspaper, breakfast (chiefly cereals with two slices of toast or maybe baked beans with or without poached eggs).

As I am unable to drive my vehicle, I have to use the public transport for all my excursions. Am also doing a steady walk in between as well for it's all helping the cause. I don't think for one minute, I am overdoing it as it has to be done for I want to walk and do things like I have done before, previously having thought that I was as fit as a person half my age. This morning—a visit to the doctor's surgery where I am to pick up more tablets to keep the body clock furthering the improvement and again to find that I have to make frequent stops.

13.00 hours I have a cheese sandwich with half an onion, then a rest, more exercises, then—what had been collecting for nearly three weeks!!!! All the JUNK MAIL!!! And my! Wasn't there some of that! I often think how much comes out of our street alone. It's been worked out that in our area, there is a ton of rubbish per household!! Now—that's a lot of waste per year!!! In the evening, a few more phone calls to make sure most who had received those Xmas cards must now be informed of my progress and I know quite a few whom I am positive will be thinking, 'I wonder how Percy is.'

January 12th

Up at 8.15 a.m. After breakfast I caught the bus to the Broadway, Debden, to do my shopping, also to visit the fish van from Grimsby with fresh fish. This lasts me well into the week with several different menus. Rest of the day—exercises, telly, wireless and of course more exercises, then my fish for my evening meal; there is still some parsley left, so what a super white sauce I enjoyed with my mashed potatoes.

January 13th

I had a lie-in this morning, without worrying about dressings; did not get up until 8.15 a.m. Before breakfast I completed roughly twenty minutes doing bed, table, settee, weights and ice-pack workouts. Through the day I roughly did two exercises every hour. In between I sorted out more old paper for removal some time by the environment collectors. The telly is going well so I can now watch in comfort and have noted down—it looks good.

January 14th

7.00 a.m. Exercises on bed for ten minutes. There seems to be quite a lot of pain on the kneecap itself. I knew it would be better when I went for paper. This was so, it seems to get set whilst I lie in bed.

I have received, from the postman this morning, a large parcel from my publishers; she has asked me to mark off in red ink any mistakes I should correct or improvements I should make in this almost final read of script. This was certainly going to help my mind from wandering in other directions. My Mrs Mopp arrived at 11.00 a.m. and she could see now the pain had come back again. I certainly was feeling on the glum side, for it was aching like the dickens. During her visit it got worse, so I decided to ring the physio at Holly House Hospital to find out if she could give me any advice. Most were busy and I could not make contact but as I have an appointment with Mr Mac for Wednesday I thought it might have settled down by then.

I phoned the publisher, who told me that the date for the book launch is now officially April 11th, so if I could get cracking on the script it was nearing the stage of going to print.

The Holly House Hospital physio rang me to give me some advice, which included administering ice packs. This would certainly help the swelling and cool it down. 'Just give me a tinkle and we will soon help if it doesn't improve,' she said.

By 13.15 hours after I had had my cream crackers, cheese and a raw onion, I had made more ice packs and wrapped them round my knee in a towel which seemed to help the situation.

My evening meal, after I had prepared it—sausages, potatoes and peas—I am afraid I did not eat all up—so, for sure, I was out of sorts!!! And brewing for something. I applied my last cold pack for the day at 21.45 hoping for a good night.

January 15th

7.00 a.m.—did some exercises on the bed. It made a big difference being able to move about without any cumbersome dressing. If only the swelling would improve.

10.00 a.m. I put my first ice pack on for the day, only keeping it on for roughly ten minutes. I then completed the proofreading of my first story about my visit to China, and had started on the Canadian trip by 12.00 hours. So time for another spell of ice pack—the weather outside had brightened up from a dull start which made me feel a bit brighter.

14.00 hours: another spell of the cold packs, then I got stuck into and completed the Canada story by just after 16.00 hours. A few phone calls between then and my evening meal completed a busy day for me. I put my final ice pack on for the day following some exercises at 20.45 hours.

January 16th

Up at 6.45 a.m. I went straightaway and got the ice packs out of the fridge for I was now kidding myself that, following the advice I had been given, an improvement was certainly on the cards and I must persevere along those lines, together with the exercises. In fact, it looks the same size as the other knee; there is just a bit of red, otherwise—colour normal. Paper, breakfast, read paper, crossword, washing eight pieces, in that order—all completed by 10.10 a.m.

Exercises rest of morning—on completion each time, a few

minutes with ice packs, continued for a time after I had my lunch break of cream crackers, cheese and onion, then a rest up until just after 14.00 hours.

Have to make myself presentable for Mr Mac at 16.40 hours.

For the life of me I still do not know why I got on a number 167 bus instead of a number 20 which would have taken me right past the Holly House Hospital.

Deciding to keep on the bus when it went down Roding Road, I got out at Buckhurst Hill Station, which even then was a good half a mile away from the hospital and nearly all up hill. The best thing—a taxi! A lady in the phone box was also inquiring for one as well. Telling her where I was going, she said, 'Would you like to share with me, as I am going that way myself?' 'Many thanks,' I said. The vehicle duly arrived, picked us up, dropped me off at Holly House Hospital with the lady not accepting any fares—just my grateful thanks.

Straight into the hospital Outpatients where the same duty nurse who looked after me a few days ago attended me with a clean and tidy-up of all the fabrics I had in place. As soon as Mr Mac saw me he said, 'We will have an x-ray done straightaway.' No, he did not like the redness all around the area where it looked pretty grim. 'There might well be a deeper infection. We will do a blood test on Friday at the Outpatients, then I want you to make an appointment for next Wednesday.'

18.30 hours I was back home via a taxi cab.

The washing I had put out on the line had already dried by the time I arrived home so I was well pleased.

January 17th

7.15 a.m. Exercises on the bed and table, finally an ice pack. Then a walk for a paper, after my breakfast. My knee seemed painful so, about four hours later, I took two more painkillers. I decided that as I was getting low on rations, I would catch the bus to the Broadway to get some fresh supplies. This all completed I was back indoors by 11.10 a.m. Quick cuppa and a few biscuits. I then concentrated on the proof-reading of the West Indies script. I had a break at 13.00 hours, then carried on until 15.45. It's reading well with very few alterations from the original script, only the vast improvements that have been made to all my missing full stops, commas, etc. The publisher lady has done a fantastic job on the punctuation.

After my evening meal, I completed some exercises, just keeping the leg moving about with quads contractions, which I know are important for strengthening the muscles. I have used those exercises since my first operation for removal of a cartilage in January 1961 on this very knee. At 21.00 hours, the knee looks pretty rough, all the red parts are certainly inflamed, with the centres turning white as though the knee's festering.

January 18th

Up at 7.15 a.m. Paper, breakfast, quick read of paper, then final read of scripts. A quick change, then bus to Holly House Hospital for my appointment with Outpatients for a blood test. Before I'd come out, I had rung Mr Mac's secretary, telling her about the concern my knee was giving me. I was to see him on Saturday at 12.00 hours.

The nurse on duty looked at it. It's dry; she applies a new dressing which seems important for it looks as if it is going to burst at any time which, as I told her, I am dreading—might well go on the bus home.

Home via Homebase, top of the road at 13.00 hours after a quick snack and few exercises, I fetched the Sharp out and completed all corrections by 16.45 hours for the West Indies story. I was very pleased that I had completed all the writing and alterations and a letter also to my insurance company—finally placing all the corrected scripts into a nice package and ready for posting tomorrow.

I left the dressing that the Outpatients nurse had put on, but prepared myself for possible eventualities with all precautions placed in my bed.

January 19th

5.00 a.m. Panic!!!! The wound has burst; it was running down my leg as I could feel it. I was so glad that I had taken the trouble to put extra protection around it, and, even then, when I had cleaned it all up, I had used up one and a half boxes of tissues (the proof in a carrier bag of used material), new dressing put in place and back in bed by 5.30 a.m.

At 7.30 a.m. I had to get up because it was throbbing so much. I had a go at my breakfast but did not seem to want to eat anything.

It was now decision time, for my plans for Saturday were now completely knocked for six. I generally do most of the shopping for the weekend, so now this has occurred, do I need to? Would Mr Mac keep me in after he had seen this pickle? I decided to go and do some, but not too much. 9.00 a.m. I caught the bus to the Broadway, made some purchases and was back at 10.45 a.m. Within a quarter of an hour I was out again and on my way for the appointment at 12.00 hours with Mr Mac. When my appointment came up (I had been called straight into Outpatients where the duty nurse had tidied the wound up and made it ready for inspection), Mr Mac looked it over and said, 'You know what this means—your holiday to New Zealand is off. It's going to be another operation—much deeper—and will be longer getting better which needs a lot of patience for all concerned.' I asked him where the infection might be—was it where he had suggested it might be before? 'Probably the outside of the bone marrow and the bone!!! Could well be in both the thigh bone and leg bone. In any case for starters, it could well be six weeks; after the operation you will be on crutches for at least a month until the wound is healed. This is important for the joints I am putting in are only temporary ones. The reason for this is because we want to make sure that the wound will heal and chiefly be free from infection. Then I'll take out the temporary ones and fit the permanent joints.' I told him confidentially about how busy a summer I was going to have with the project I was involved with, hoping to have my first book published, also giving him the date April 11th as the launch at the bookshop in Epping. The Outpatients nurse tidied me up as Mr Mac tells me: 'I want you to come in for the operation next Thursday.' On the way out I saw several staff who wanted to know when I was coming to see them again. When I told them I would be coming to see them next Thursday, one said, 'You do this on purpose!'

Back home, I carried on with all the rest of my Saturday duties, but was glad that I had posted the parcel to the publisher lady. I was hoping to get in touch with my pal in Somerset to tell him that my holiday to New Zealand was off. I know he would be disappointed.

Sunday, January 20th

Had a bit of a lie-in for the whole leg felt uncomfortable. So it was 8.00 a.m. before I ventured out to get the paper. I walked there and back with the whole knee wrapped with dressings and tissues, finally taped all round with a piece of plastic—this in turn taped with Microtape.

I knew something was up as soon as I got back in the house and, after taking off the old dressings, there it was—all oozing down my leg. So more tidying up with dressings from my supplies with a final layer of tissues held down with Microtape. This then sorted me out for the rest of the day.

I started and completed several chores that I would normally have left until the next day, including several pieces of washing, and as there was a good blow going on outside, knew this would be worthwhile. All change at 14.00 hours for it was pouring with rain by then so all the washing and myself beat a hasty retreat with quite a lot almost dry.

Just before I went to bed I put a clean dressing on for the night, after giving it a close inspection. With nothing much changed during the day, my word it did look fiery and ferocious! This is how I have described it in my diary and now as I am taking those notes down I have looked at the definition of ferocious in the dictionary I keep close by. It says, 'Savage, fierce'!!! and this I might say is very apt for I recall quite clearly how at the time it was just that. Time 23.00 hours.

January 21st

7.00 a.m. went for a paper with the dressing still in place for it seemed secure and without any leakage. This might have been because I had kept the whole leg in the one position all night. I am pretty sure this was why I hardly saw any discharge when I went to change it after I returned with the paper.

After I had got things shipshape again and after breakfast about 9.30 a.m. I managed to get through to my pal in Somerset, telling him the bad news that I would not be able to make our holiday in New Zealand.

I phone my Mrs Mopp, asking her to purchase more tissues and bring them along with her, because I was now using them again as if there was no tomorrow. Typed a letter for my own doctor explaining to him the whys and wherefores as to my going back into hospital.

January 22nd

Same sort of day as the day before.

January 23rd

Very similar, only that when I got up to go for the paper, I sat down to change the dressings only to find that the second bump had now burst and had been discharging as well!!!!! What a mess!!!

January 24th

Up at 6.20 a.m. The second bump has now formed a hole and blood and pus is oozing through. I completed all my phone calls last night, so now all I have to do is finish my packing.

Taxi took me and delivered me to Holly House Hospital at 11.15 a.m. This was mighty strange for not only was it the same ward that I was in at Xmas but also the same room, no 151. It seems as if the hospital is full up and, during the rest of the morning and afternoon, my operation looked as if it was going to be put off. Mr Mac came in at 13.00 hours and asked if there were any questions and asked me if I would sign the consent forms, then telling me that, after my op, I would have to make do with crutches for some time. Mr Dodd soon arrived wishing me well. I had not had anything to eat or drink for my operation was down for the afternoon and then later postponed to 22.00 hours. I said to the sister bringing me this news, 'What? 10.00 at night!' It was then decided that I should be given a round of toast and a pot of tea, for it had now been several hours since I had been fed and watered. After my wash and shave at 19.00 hours, the senior sister came in and said that due to hold-ups—no operation today— postponed until Saturday afternoon. It was not long before Mr Mac came in, and apologised, saying that there were complications in the theatre.

January 25th

I had a pretty good night, considering, and was awake at 5.00 a.m. After an early morning cuppa and breakfast, which I enjoyed, for it was the most I had eaten since this time yesterday, I went for a walk along the corridor and renewed friendships with staff, who I had considered unlikely to be seeing again for a long time, but now seemingly about to be long-term friends! During the morning and afternoon, my telephone was in use quite frequently; most wanted to know how I was feeling after my operation, each had to be told that owing to unforeseen circumstances, it had been put off until Saturday afternoon. I had kept my dressing on all day, since the night staff had changed it quite early and I recall there was some vile looking stuff. It was changed later at approximately 22.00 hours for a new one.

January 26th

As early as 4.30 a.m. I called the night nurse as it was discharging and the dressing was changed. I was so pleased that today might see the last of this business—as I was beginning to wonder if this would ever come to an end for it seemed relentless in its attempts to conjure up this offensive matter. When I inquire about this situation, I am told—it is restricted and there's no need to do any worrying.

I was due to go down to theatre at 17.00 hours and as I had been prepared for this some two hours before, I was pleased when the porters came along to take me down for I was nearly asleep.

In the recovery room, for some strange reason, I was in another country with all the staff of a dark skin. I wanted to cough and spit but was told by one very large black nurse, 'You can't do that here, only into this tissue.'!!! One hallucination, the other reality. I have also noted that it feels as if I have a ton weight attached to my leg. The nurse in charge when I got back to 151 told me that what I had attached to leg were braces which were to stop me from bending it and to keep it straight at all times.

January 27th

I have officially named this room 151!!ACTION ROOM!!!! For without a shadow of doubt—and I am pretty positive with my thinking—on the different occasions I have been in this room, action of some sort or another occurs. So what sort of tales can this room tell of patients who have frequented its four walls, perhaps even of ordinary people when it was a private house; was this the room which a ghost was supposed to have been linked to? And what goes on in here now whilst I am laying defenceless in this bed?

I had several cups of tea in the night at the times when I was allowed painkillers and I was thankful when they started working.

I ate my breakfast of toast and cereals and was now beginning to feel the bandage which was wrapped around the knee, above and below, and this was no ordinary one for it was a crepe one. 10.45 a.m. the nurses changed the sheets and I take this chance to have a good look at the brace as well, which encircled the whole package. I was to carry this around with me for perhaps four weeks????

The x-ray department sent up the machine together with the lady operator, who managed to take some frames in various positions whilst I was lying on the bed with my trusty pole overhead—me a true monkey in these manoeuvres whilst this was taking place. Within a quarter of an hour, the photos were developed and placed in the holder for Mr Mac to see. Mind you I had a look before they went in, after the young lady had said, 'They are very good.' I agreed but was not sure what was what.

Mr Mac called in about 12.00 hours and wanted to see his handiwork, so the bandage was removed. My—it did look a mess but a tidy one. He warned, 'What you must do is keep the leg as straight as possible at all times. When you get out of bed, be careful that you always get assistance as you really will need help then.'

The physio called in later to say that exercises are only to be from side to side for starters. That's easy contractions—this will keep the leg moving before the important ones begin at a later date. During the day I have had very little pain and have managed to do my regular duties quite well, have also eaten all my meals—including dinner which was a salad, dessert apple pie and custard.

I had a late-night drink of hot chocolate and later still I had a sleeping tablet. Lights out at 21.00 hours.

January 28th

6.00 a.m. The night sister is around with antibiotics after early morning cuppa. I begin to have more confidence in moving my leg around but as it is almost an impossibility to bend or straighten I am only slowly acquiring confidence that all parts had been connected up again correctly. This is a feeling that is difficult to put down on paper for it is something that keeps nagging—whenever your knee is opened up (and now this is the fourth time)! So I am well pleased that I can wriggle my toes. Nurse came along to walk me very ungraciously to the toilet which I found most uncomfortable because, since I had to keep the leg straight, it was more than difficult to sit down. It was fortunate that I had the raising piece fitted so this eased the pain quite a bit.

As I was walking with crutches and only able to walk on the one leg, or rather hop, I was glad when both the number 1 and 2 physios came in to show me how I should use the crutches by taking me to the door and back, I have marked down: *very unsteady—must improve.*

Mr Mac called in at 14.00 hours, had a look at the inside of the brace and said, 'It's most important that you keep your weight off the repaired leg and, whatever you do, do not lift the whole leg. Oh, and the drain can come out of the wound now.' (It had been draining into the jam jar attached to frame of bed.) He also told Sister that, as the right arm is painful, change it to the left one to get the antibiotics in.

Ate all my food, usual practice—ordered the day before, received more phone calls and sent a few out.

It was later when the night shift had taken over that I had the drain removed, for there had been a slight discharge since the order for its removal was sanctioned, so being positive, sister had used her logic and kept it in until the smallest of milligrams had been accounted for.

January 29th

I had a pretty good night; in fact at 6.10 a.m. I had some tablets, early morning cuppa at 7.15 a.m. then after breakfast at 8.10 a.m. I went to the toilet, helped along by the nurse in charge of me, remembering no weight on repaired leg, lightly on heel, the same as the toe, these measures to avoid complications. I have marked down—bloody awkward!

10.30 a.m. Two physios arrive and help me to just outside the door and back, must have taken ten minutes; was glad to get back to bed, have marked down—bloody painful!

12.00 hours—regular time for jab in the tummy to prevent foreign bodies getting involved with me again. Lunch arrives—cream crackers, all sorts of cheeses, tomato and a raw onion. Had a couple of visitors whilst the maintenance man had come in to do some repairs, as well as replace a light bulb.

At 19.30 hours, the drip which I had had attached to me since the operation was removed. This had been giving me trouble for some time, and a new one was fitted. Had painkillers later.

January 30th

There has been a slight disaster, for the drip had been leaking, so the sheets had to be changed, this was after the night staff had been almost clear of their duties.

After my breakfast and, telling the nurse that I wanted to use the toilet, it was this time, the one and only, that I got muddled up with which leg I should start walking with. The nurse almost shouted, 'You have to hop, Percy, on your good leg!!!'

Back on the bed after I had found most of the walking about exhausting, it feels all right. With practice, I find that I am getting more used to avoiding the thing I most want to avoid, and that is to put the whole weight down onto the floor. At 17.45 hours, the antibiotics are to go into my arm, and the nurse is finding it difficult to get it going. This I had witnessed with several patients on my earlier travels, but it was not long before all was well and successful. At 19.30 hours, Sister had called in to see how my right arm was. Other nurses had reported it inflamed, so she decided to put a hot Kaolin poultice on with a crepe bandage placed round with the trusty Micropore tape keeping it in place.

Mr Mac called in at 21.00 hours, asked the sister to release all the bandages wrapped round the leg—and, my word, were there some yards of crepe, then, looking at his work, said, 'Looks fine.' He also took a quick look at the x-rays, then told the sister to replace the large bandage with a light dressing.

This is applied shortly after he has gone but with a gauze-type of material directly over the steel stitches with a light dressing directly under the brace—which I don't believe I have described before; it goes from the top of my thigh down to the curvature of my ankle and leg. It's made up of two halves with Velcro straps as fixings, and, of course, now that all the crepe bandage has been taken off, has to be readjusted. The canes inside make the whole brace a combined piece of excellent splint appliance. What a difference it makes without the crepe bandage, it feels ten times lighter, so this has cheered me up enormously.

January 31st

As I do not want to get out of bed too often, I found I was using the bottle more often to relieve myself, in fact frequently, owing to the amount of fluids I was drinking, no doubt.

6.30 a.m. Antibiotics drip and Vac Flo—the latter the correct name for the goodies that are pumped into my arm through this attachment fixed to the nerve on the back of my wrist. Shortly after this an early morning cuppa, breakfast at 8.15 a.m. Have had extra baked beans this morning. I dare say the chef knows that I enjoy them.

8.50 a.m. Went to toilet, managed all the important items; the male nurse who was looking after me also took off the Kaolin poultice that had been applied last night but, unfortunately, it had made very little difference despite my singing its praises last night when sister was applying it, telling her that when we were children it used to go on in big dollops to cure any inflammatory injury, redness, swelling, or pain. Why had it not been successful, you might well ask!!! It had travelled from the staff room, so the heat had almost gone before it had been applied, then bandaged to seal the remaining warmth in. As the sister remarked at the time, 'We'll give it a try, Percy.' When I saw her again, I said, 'We can't win.' Have not seen the physio this morning but am sure I am on the list for early afternoon. This was the case, I was to find out.

12.00 hours—tummy and Vac Flo injections. Win, the patient across the corridor has had an accident and is leaking blood, and, like me, mislays or drops the red buzzer (emergency bell), so would I oblige her? 'Certainly,' I replied.

It was not long after my lunch had disappeared and my nap was due when the physiotherapist appeared, this time with a metal wheelie frame which seemed to give me a bit more balance, but no sooner had I told her this, than wham! Fortunately she was nearby and so was the wall, otherwise I would have toppled over. It looked as if you could never turn a frame over but I learnt this wasn't so. Mind you, it might have been because it had two wheels attached to the front. Realising that I must make progress, I said I would persevere with the lift, hop and step order. I was to get this wrong many times, but then I was to learn that I would have to do this for several weeks, so I must be more constructive with my concentration.

A letter off to one of my cricket pals in the Midlands to let him know of my situation.

Before my evening meal, the day sister on duty came in to fix a new entry box into the vein to get the fluids in and in doing so it broke!!! So the duty doctor had to be called in to attach a new one; both the sachets were emptied by 18.10 hours, just in time for our dinner to arrive. It was no discomfort to have them in when eating a meal but of course it was much better without. Especially as it was beef pie, various veg and, for dessert, plum pudding. Again! (I have marked 'again' in my diary so I must have had it before, perhaps at lunch time.)

This sister on duty, if she ever reads this, will know that I am referring to her. For some reason I always managed to get her name wrong even though we were hardly strangers to one other. It's now ten years since we first made acquaintance; I can only say how sorry I am because I know it offends her.

She had gone off duty just after 21.00 hours but, when she came in to see how the entry box was faring and to say goodnight, it was way past her scheduled time for finishing and I can assure anyone interested in reading this little piece that I refer to many such dedicated sisters, staffs and nurses, in exactly the same circumstances.!!! TIME 23.15 hours.

February 1st

6.15 a.m. The night sister gets me on the drip again, this time with two fresh sachets. By 7.00 a.m. both are empty. As I have been watching this operation I notice the staff turn this small tap on and off, and for other patients likewise. I do this myself while there is some fluid left in the plastic pipe because if it's completely drained off it sometimes results in an air blockage, making it difficult to start up again. So if I am able to assist in any way that's going to improve my lot, don't hold me back!!!!!

Early morning cuppa—7.20 a.m. Then, just after 8.00 a.m. breakfast arrives. I mention that I have eaten every bit—if so it would have been cereals, poached eggs (2), baked beans, toast (2), and marmalade.

The day nurse arrives to change the linen and takes me for a hop and trot to the toilet. She also attends to the DVT stockings which she puts on in a different way to others but they are in the right place (vent holes) despite my wriggling and fidgeting about. They will be lucky if they stop in that position all day.

11.30 a.m. Another nurse is having trouble too with the antibiotics going into my wrist I have marked down: 'It has all gone in but blood is being pressured.' (Can't account for this remark!) It might be something to do with the Vac Flo which has been removed. No doubt staff with knowledge will understand what I have been going through. Physio arrives for a walk—11.45. 12.00 hours CC arrive with cheeses, a tomato and onion, dessert is rice pudding. One of the management team came in saying she was off for the weekend and wished me a happy birthday—wow!—for Sunday the 3rd.

17.45 hours Mr Mac comes in, brace is undone, also dressing. He said, 'It looks fine. I think it's nearly time we put you on the machine. We must do this to make sure that when the new joints are fitted the whole knee is nice and supple to receive them, so getting them off to a good start is a must.'

Looking at my wrist, he says, 'It should fade and gradually disappear, for you can take your antibiotics orally now.' He tells the nurse how many, and times are sorted out too. The dressing is then replaced and as I am beginning to get the hang of the brace equipment, I help to put it back together again, and, as it was a new nurse on the block, she appreciated this.

Saturday, 2nd February

I have had a good night—tablets at 6.45 a.m. The night staff have been on duty for the second night on the trot—no it's not unusual but this particular staff nurse does not usually do nights—I will have to ask her. Like all the nursing staff, if the pressure is on, patient care seems to come before domestic duties!!! (Shall I say the majority of cases?) Mind you, now I have said that I can recall when I first came in back in September, there was a nurse on duty permanent nights and still doing it—dedication and knowledge.

Today is also when the weekend Mrs Moppses arrive, same type of girls as the weekday ones. These three girls—again they are equally jolly, friendly and busy. Do they rabbit!! As they are audible, usually putting the worlds to rights, I call them the three pluses. Have completed all my duties before 9.00 a.m. The linen is changed and I'm reading the paper when I can hear the sergeant major about—I often picture this physiotherapist in the uniform of a WRAF Sergeant. Proper no-nonsense type: 'Now come along, please, this will not do, move along. Do you want to get better or don't you!' A type of strength she innocently disguises but she is very proficient and gentle like the day physio ladies. 'Hello, not you again!' 'Yes, I am afraid so,' I replied, asking her if she had any orders to put me on the CPM. 'No, I have not heard it mentioned, but I will make inquiries because Mr Mac will want to push on with your exercises.'

Anyhow, we had a walk along the corridor. I was finding that I really needed the frame, and regular stops; after some eight hops I was glad to stop and lean against a door jamb to recover from the exertion—to my knowledge I had not done any hopping since school days when it was hop-skip-and-jump!!! My—that was a long time ago—and if I recall I used to fall over even then—and that was with two good legs, but very short though!

Had visitors in the afternoon. Sue, the retired staff nurse who is such a good friend knows exactly what I am going through—as no doubt she has worked with hundreds of cases like mine, always offering good advice.

All my meals had been consumed and enjoyed—but I have realised that in-between snacks are temptations that must be avoided—I don't know how long my stay is going to be but I want to go back home, within a few pounds of what I weighed when I came here.

It was well into the late evening and late-night drinks had come together with a biscuit or two—when I asked the night staff nurse if she would come and have a chat with me. I asked her if she had heard whether I was to go on the CPM machine because Mr Mac had spoken about it yesterday, saying it was important that I make as much progress as I can by using the CPM to keep the knee exercised and supple. 'Leave it to me, Percy. I'll make a note of this and to be sure it will be sorted for your good self tomorrow.'

One of the staff nurses has a birthday as well tomorrow for I know that it's hers—but pretty sure she does not know it's mine. It's just another day for me except I am just another year older!!! The date is February 3rd.

February 3rd

7.50 a.m. Early morning cuppa, found a few Rich Tea biscuits—then I could hear several voices coming along the corridor. Within a few minutes, in marched all the night staff together with a few day ones, all giving me a chorus of 'Happy Birthday' together with birthday cards. I had to cover my head under the sheets for indeed I was shedding a tear or two. Breakfast, extra baked beans as well.

By 9.40 a.m. all my dailies had been long done and I'm reading the paper when the sergeant major in charge of physio came in with other nurses—another chorus of 'Happy Birthday' with more cards. I couldn't believe it—I had never been treated like this before—physio says, 'See you later, orders are—you start the CPM machine this morning.' Sure thing 11.00 a.m. the machine arrives and I stay on until 12.00 hours just keeping it at twenty-five degrees—mind you, you could soon get carried away for it is such a soothing action, that if you are not keeping an eye open, you would quickly doze off. But, fortunately, I have a few answers left to solve in the crossword, so am keeping awake doing this. More visitors just before lunch break—they had been with me for some ten minutes, when both said, 'What, is it your birthday, Perc?' and I knew them quite well.

12.00 hours. Sunday roast, baked, boiled potatoes, various vegetables, plum pudding and custard. Whew! I had a walk along the corridor; later back in 151 made a few phone calls, also had some incoming ones as well. 15.00 hours—another surprise. About ten nurses came in with a birthday cake. Another chorus of 'Happy Birthday' and was told afterwards that all the other rooms were joining in as well. Again, I gave each one a special hug because nothing like this had ever happened to me before or is maybe likely to ever again (I hoped it might occur but not in hospital!). Up to 15.30 hours for roughly about an hour, I was on the machine—nothing excessive, up to forty degrees—just to keep the leg moving.

There had been some exciting cricket, for England had beaten India by five runs—so guessed that my pal in Somerset had been watching it, for he has Sky telly and would be at home. I rang him asking him if he had enjoyed the match: 'What a game,' he said, 'with Freddie Flintoff taking the last Indian wicket—Srinath's.' I told him what a day I had been having to celebrate my birthday. I still had other cards to arrive— one delivered by a nurse who arrived with her coat almost wet through—as she said special delivery—a big hug and left also two pressies for me. This was Pultzer—so named for being so enterprising.

18.00 hours—scampi, chips, peas, carrots and dessert plum pudding.

My good friend Derrick arrived from the nearby housing estate and I told him about all the excitement I had had for my birthday and of course I gave him a small portion of the cake which I know he enjoyed.

Bed at 22.45 hours have noted down—tired and weary— owing to all the excitement.

February 4th

6.30 a.m. Night staff along with trolley—have been informed that I should take the pills with my breakfast, which arrived at 8.10 a.m.

As I had collected some red patches on my backside, I had been wearing what are termed 'patches' to relieve the rawness and reduce the pain—the staff removed them saying that the area is much improved. Also a back wash—with a good rub down with the towel—the modern towelling off as you might not be aware is with gentle dabs over the wet parts—this a modern method for drying; I know which I prefer.

At 9.20, I was back on the bed after getting back into the brace!!! Knackered!!!

It was not long before the physiotherapist arrives; as you

Happy Birthday Percy, have a good time
love from Sarah

Happy Birthday love Joan x

Dear Percy Have a nice one. Enjoy yourself
Camille

To Percy Many Happy Returns Love Jane

Happy Birthday Percy Many happy returns of the day. Take care
Tracy

Dear Percy Hope you have a lovely day. Many happy returns.
Gemma

Wishing you a memorable 74th Birthday. Best Wishes
Marion

Happy 75th Birthday Percy

A very Happy 74th Birthday Percy! Remember - you are only as young as old as you feel!!! With love
Rudi Velter

Dear Percy All the best for you but you know that England will go down against the GERMANS!!!

"IT'S YOUR BIRTHDAY!"

Percy Have a good day. Many Happy Returns.
Nora

Have a good day. Many happy returns
Diane M.

Happy Birthday Percy. Is it your 16th?
Love Sylvia

can see very little peace! Straight on the CPM, then whilst this passive movement was in operation I had three visitors arrive who kept me laughing until the time the lunch arrived, and then as there was heaps of cheese and biscuits, they tucked in as well—they left at 12.40 with both visitors and patient in a very happy state of mind—Tony and John, both Old Chigwellians and Tony, the post.

Early afternoon I was taken for a walk along the corridor—then 14.40 on the CPM. Mr Mac called in at 15.00 hours—had a look at the wound. I pointed out to him the swelling that had appeared on the outside part of the thigh, his reply: 'It's muscle, should sort itself out.' He also asked me what degrees I had reached so far, as he reminded me that he wants the knee to be nice and supple for the next operation. I replied, 'Fifty degrees.'

Soon after 18.00 hours, dinner arrives—chicken, new potatoes, calabrese; mixed fruit as the dessert, grapes, slices of apple, pear, pineapple and peaches. Late drink arrives 20. 45 hours.

February 5th

6.00 a.m. Medical trolley on the move so you always know which sister is on duty most times. Not only is the medical trolley making an early start but the early morning cuppa. 7.05, followed at 7.50 a.m. by breakfast.

8.25 a.m.—out to toilet. This morning I could have had an accident, for as I was having my shave and leaning on the towel rail, with my left arm, the bracket came away from the wall with the weight I was transferring on it. Fortunately, as I went down on the floor my repaired leg was jarred but no damage done. The nurse who was changing the sheets quickly came to my rescue and soon dusted me down saying, 'How did you come to do that?' Like I told her, 'It's pretty difficult when you are trying not to put weight on the foot not to lean on the wall or something for support.' At the time I know I was standing on my heel, the left elbow was lying on the towel rail, and my other arm, the right one, was holding the razor whilst looking in the mirror!!!

Of course, word quickly got around that Perc was trying to break out!!! But the rail was quickly repaired by the maintenance staff, within a half hour of sister reporting it.

I went on the CPM at 11.00 a.m. and stayed on for an hour and reached fifty-two degrees without any bother, for after a tumble like I'd had, you wonder if you have undone the good work that you have already committed yourself to.

This morning also I have had a fair sized parcel arrive. I was very surprised to find it contained three cricket books but with no message from anyone. So I had to guess whom it might be from. From any one of ten people who might be thoughtful enough to get me reading about the great *Brian Johnson—A Hundred Years of Test Cricket at Lords* or *Jim Laker*.

After lunch I completed some letters and made a few phone calls, just after our afternoon cuppa I had more visitors. I went on the CPM for an hour between 16.15 hours and 17.45 hours. I did make a mistake here because I had been told to give it about an hour gradually building it up to what the physiotherapist had asked me to work to. This afternoon for some reason, I stayed on another half an hour. Perhaps I was too busy wondering who could have sent me such a nice birthday present; it was two days late, I know but it's always the thought that counts and that's always important to me.

There was a call I wanted to make a fair distance away but, as my brain was not functioning all that well, I decided to leave it until tomorrow.

After late night drinks and just before lights out, final pills for the day, including my sleeping one.

February 6th

Did not have a bad night.

6.15 a.m. Trolley on the move with all patients' needs moving along combined with the chink of the keys which are faithfully locked up and unlocked for each stop of this vehicle!!! How many turns of the locks, during the course of its three journeys daily along the corridor, could be anyone's guess—and of course it is also well equipped with emergency equipment. My bottom is also inspected this morning by the staff nurse; by my reckoning today will be my fourteenth day here since I arrived on the 24th January.

Back in bed at 9.15 a.m. after doing all my chores—trying to make the telephone call that I wanted to make yesterday. I tried at regular intervals until I eventually got through at 10.15 a.m. Our discussion was about the launch date of my book that was being published and I was telling the publisher of my progress, and how it might well affect the date we all have in mine—but would keep her informed.

The CPM machine was waiting for me when I had completed all my business, saying to the physiotherapist, 'The office is now closed and ready for work of a different kind.' Gave the machine a quick burst up to sixty degrees, turning if off at 11.55 a.m.

Afternoon I went for my usual walk along the corridor—beg your pardon—hop, step, stop and lean against a door jamb—yes, the same one, only about fifteen yards!!! And that knackered me!!! Of course, the physiotherapist is holding my arm. Straight on the CPM: our aim this afternoon was sixty degrees and to hold it there. Which when I was taken off later, told her this was my achieved goal—holding for some ten minutes.

Dinner 18.00 hours—chicken, roast potatoes, three sorts of vegetables, dessert is apple pie and custard. Mr Mac called in at 18.45 hours, has a look at the wound saying, 'It looks as if the wound is healing well.' He says, 'I would like to keep the stitches in until your blood count is back to normal, perhaps a few more weeks.' He reminds me again that they are only temporary joints that are attached at the moment. 'There are times,' I tell him, 'when I am at a loss as to the reasoning behind this.' As he explains again, for only the second occasion, all will be well once the infection is cleared up completely and everything is fine to carry out the final operation. I had heard through the hospital grapevine that another patient in similar circumstances might well be going home for a few weeks.

February 7th

Had a pretty good night—trolley on the move at 5.45 a.m. This morning it seems very busy already for all the rooms I am told are occupied. All jobs attended to and back on the bed by 9.00 a.m. Reading the paper, post arrives, with one from an old pal in Suffolk who asks me if I have enjoyed reading the books. 'Well, I'm blowed.' He would have been one of the last I would have thought to list as having sent such beautiful books—because I know he is suffering some mighty poor health himself! There you go—it takes all sorts.

CPM machine from 10.45 a.m. to nearly 12.00 hours.

Had a couple of letters to finish so it was not until 15.20 that the nurse came to take me for a walk or hop—still a struggle, have gone a bit further today for I am sure it's twenty yards there and back to the entrance to Room 151—then on to the machine. CPM for an hour—up to sixty degrees—felt all right.

Derrick arrives and stays for nearly an hour. He always seems interested in what is going on in almost every room and have introduced him to several patients; for this I know he is highly chuffed.

One thing about today: it is nice to be indoors for it has been raining nearly all day. I enjoyed my dinner—chicken pie, calabrese, mash, sweetcorn, dessert is apple crumble and custard. One of my final jobs for the day was to console one of the new nurses, as she seemed mighty upset because a patient was quite ill and needed a lot of her attention. I tried to explain to her how important it was for the patient to get involved with her—the nurse. I put it quite bluntly to her that it is one of the most important parts of her job—to hold the patient's hand for as long as she thinks fit, for there is nothing more reassuring than for a nurse to calm, soothe, reason and stay calm as the tension builds; never desert your post for that's the last thing you should do, unless you have to say, 'Well I must go for I have to prepare the family meal,' or a really valid excuse. 'Cheer her up, that's your job and the sister will chalk you up some high marks for doing this.' The nurse looked at me in amazement!!! Am sure it worked.

Late night drink—hot chocolate, then before lights out—my sleeping pill.

February 8th

I have several names for the nurses and there are a few who, I am sure, know why I call them such and such names. One such nurse I call Shotgun Annie, for when you talk to her, her replies are as if they have been fired at breakneck speed straight from the hip—again a very dedicated nurse and quite often using her own judgement—counts for long years of experience.

Early movers on duty so if anyone thought they were going to have a bit of a lie-in—they had another think coming for the trolley was on the move at 6.00 a.m. Early morning cuppa—7.25 a.m. Breakfast at 8.00 a.m., no baked beans this morning—I could hear there were a few problems, so I did not want to pile on the pressure.

It's quite regular now to have more and more nurses coming from the Agency. This morning I have one looking after me and it appears a strong certainty that these nurses are trained to dab your back, to dry it after the final part of a wash and brush-up is out of the way. I said to her, 'Don't worry, you give it a good hard rub.' Am not sure if she understood. In any case it made not the slightest difference.

The physio arrived at 10.20 a.m. First of all, a walk along the corridor: I suppose it is now the length of a cricket pitch that I walk. No, don't get me wrong—that's there and back—you have to remember that I am still hopping on the one leg and am thankful about the frequent stops that I have during that time. Time is immaterial really but I daresay that it takes just under ten minutes to go there and come back.

Straight on the CPM until 12.00 hours.

Lunch CC: various cheeses, tomato, raw onion; am pretty sure that the food I am now eating is good for the figure and helping to keep my weight attended to. If there is going to be any increase then it won't be for want of trying on my part to keep it within reason. Another patient, Jennie has now gone after having a hip replacement. There have been so many, for the room opposite has had four different patients since I arrived here. Each one I got to know quite well with names and addresses changing hands but know over many years of doing this, very few of these take off into lasting friendships. One person who was here the same time as me seven years ago, I still keep in touch with, for my word, she was and still is a cheerful person with her illness and bravery. I call myself a very lucky chap when I think how her body has been pulled about. She could write a book herself—for her it's long-term.

After lunch, I had a visit from the maintenance telly man to put the picture right. No problem and soon sorted out. Started a letter to Joe, the chap who sent me the books, telling him how much I appreciated them and found them fascinating reading. It's strange how easy I find it to write a letter and I'm able to do it without referring to the large *Longman Synonym Dictionary* that I have at home. Mind you, there is a super person here who has been such a help to me with a problem if one crops up.

At 15.00 hours, you will never guess, but I am being supplied with a new chart as the old book is full up.

At 15.45 hours, I am taken for a walk, then at 16.05 a.m. put on the CPM. My friend Derrick arrived at 17.00 hours, just as I had been taken off the CPM so I asked him a few cricket questions that I wanted to help prepare for a few of my cricket pals in the form of a quiz question and answer sheet. He did not know any of the five I had put together but he enjoyed it.

Dinner at 18.00 hours. One of my favourites—scampi, peas, chips and dessert is treacle pudding. 19.00 hours—Mr Mac called in. Dressing off: 'The wound looks good. Tomorrow we can have a few stitches out, perhaps two or three,' he told the nurse taking all the notes. Crutches were also mentioned during this conversation.

February 9th

It seemed as if every room along the Cedar Ward corridor was in need of help at 6.00 hours, 'odd being as it's Saturday'. This is surprising but knowing who the sister is (important to get on with it) it's best to leave nothing to worry about with when changeover is due if an emergency arises. Only one of the waitresses on duty—I told her I would give her a hand if I could walk a bit better. What a smile though—this made me feel heaps better. All chores completed by 9.00 a.m. Am informed that the staff nurse in charge of me is going to remove the stitches. As there was a hold-up, it was decided to take me for a walk, then the CPM; by that time the staff would be free to take out the steel ones but leave the wax ones. I said to her when she started, 'I don't see the point of leaving them in. Why couldn't they come out?' I had now cast some doubt in the staff nurse's mind as she said, 'I will go and ask the sister.' This was done almost straightaway but the answer came back to say they are to stop in. I had reached seventy degrees on the machine, so was quite pleased with the morning's occupations. In the afternoon I lost count of all the visitors who came to see me. However, everyone who called went away with the knowledge that I had still to undergo another operation. At one time, there were seven people in with me and, of course, which is only natural, one of the friends had to use the loo. I told him where it was and not to worry about the raising piece!! All of a sudden the panic buzzer shrieked out and he was not aware who it was who had set this off, for he had naturally thought that this was the pull which operates the cistern. Not so—three nurses dived in to find out what Percy was up to this time!!! My! We all had a good laugh about this. He certainly saw the funny side of it and it was only when the nurses came in that he realised what he had done. Francis, his wife, who is a midwife, was, I can assure you, totally in fits, for she straightaway knew what he had done!!!

I had more books delivered by this company, so there was no need for me to watch the telly too often now; as far as I was concerned, this was all knowledge material and all beneficial to the grey cells. After they had gone, I had my walk. Then I was put on the CPM until dinner time when I had reached again seventy degrees.

Beef stroganoff, Brussels, mash, peas, apple and plum strudel!! Whew!!! You could quite understand the 'whew!' if you had witnessed the meal before I started, as I have marked down. Late night drink, then later—painkillers and ST.

February 10th

Again—early start with trolley on the move before 6.00 a.m. The waitress on duty (this one I call 'my little nicotine girl'— am not sure if she likes a fag) is on the ball pretty quick especially with the early cuppas.

All the duties and chores completed by 9.00 a.m. which included a thorough knocking about with the staff nurse who held the drying towel. Yes, she had been around for a few years! Like me, she knew how to handle them. That's all I say to most of them: 'You wait until my legs are better, then you might not be able to avoid dodging me.' This same staff nurse said just to cheer me up, 'When the physio arrives, you are to use the crutches this morning.' I said, 'Oh no, I am dreading them!' as I had seen Lawrence using them and knew he didn't like them. Still, he got used to them eventually. I did not want to do this, but if it was going to be to my advantage, then I had better wait and see.

When the physio arrived—sure thing—just after 10.30 a.m. crutches arrived with her. I had a go with them for a few minutes but as the physio said at the time, 'We have done enough with them. I'll put you on the machine.' Had orders for it to go to eighty degrees. Over the hour I reached seventy degrees and that was a struggle.

12.00 hours—I had a toasted cheese sandwich with lettuce and tomato.

Afternoon at 15.40 hours, I was back in the frame hopping and leaning against the frames of various doors on the way down and back in the corridor. Another physio on duty and am pretty sure she has not put many patients on the CPM but, after a lesson or two from me, she soon got the hang of it. Up to seventy-five degrees and holding so I was pleased.

My friend Derrick called in and stayed for twenty minutes, telling me it's a decent day with very little rain. Dinner at 18.15—scampi, peas and chips. Later hot chocolate, PK and ST.

February 11th

Trolley on the move at 6.00 a.m. Shot Gun Annie is also on duty—all the observations quickly taken care of. Early morning cuppa arrives, then at 7.20 a.m. the RD arrives to take a blood sample. Breakfast at 7.50 a.m. and by 8.30 a.m. all jobs had been completed including a change of bedlinen.

9.10 a.m. Physio came along and left a nurse in charge of me. This was not unusual for it was just a question of making sure that I was accompanied by a senior nurse or the like. I much prefer the frame and it's the wheel-less version for, as I have mentioned, the wheelie one goes too quickly for me in my state of health. Back on the CPM I reached seventy-five degrees, completing this task at 11.45 a.m. Lunch back on the CC, cheese and tomato. During this period, Mr Mac called in, had a look at the wound, saying, after reading my chart, 'We will have the rest of the stitches out today, it's looking good.'

I had been in touch with my insurance today for an assurance about my situation. The lady at the other end of the line, helping me with my enquiries said, 'Everything is okay.' They are now waiting for another follow-up report on Mr McAuliffe's latest consultation.

During this afternoon, I had several visitors. During one of the visits, the senior staff came in with a couple of Philippino nurses who are working in the hospital. It appears they are fully trained nurses but it was to their advantage that, even if they knew how to remove stitches, to learn, not necessarily a better method, but one that was proven here. No machine this afternoon, by orders of the physio and Mr Mac I suppose.

On investigating where the stitches had been, it did look red and raw and again. I said to myself, 'To think it has all got to be opened up again!' Yet it was nice to acknowledge that all the pieces from this major op had all been connected again properly.

At dinner I thought it might have been a bit special according to the menu sheet!!! It was entitled Chicken Princess. It was not very different to the usual cooked one—just tarted up a little. Enjoying the veggies and new potatoes that came along as well. Plum pudding was my dessert.

February 12th

5.45 a.m. Drug trolley on the move. 7.15 early morning cuppa. All observations completed. No toast with my poached eggs when breakfast arrived at 8.15 a.m. Word sent down to chef in charge—Percy has no toast: four minutes and it was sent in—how can I ever repay those waitresses! Everything completed by 9.15 a.m. including change of stockings and legs creamed as well. This was a request of mine, for I felt they were getting on the rough side but fortunately my backside was doing well and was not having any problems considering I am now going into my eighteenth day with very little time to get up and move about. Certainly, I was not bed-bound but spent a lot of the day lying in bed.

The physiotherapist arrives and is considerate for she could see that I was in the last stages of an important letter I wanted to get off by the midday post—one I had started as soon as I awoke. Explaining this to her, 'No problem,' she said. 10.30 a.m. to 11.40 a.m. on the CPM keeping and holding seventy-five degrees.

After lunch, at 14.00 hours, Lawrence and Eric arrived and stayed for a couple of hours; both of them are a great laugh and I as well as the staff and other patients enjoyed their company. I have jotted down—a smashing time with them and was sorry to see them go as I am sure the staff were as well. I did go on the CPM for just over the hour up to seventy-five degrees.

18.00 hours—shepherds pie, calabrese, carrots with apple pie and custard. Later I made a phone call to a good friend of mine, who has also been involved with hospitals. But his worries are his eyes. During the war he was involved with the resistance in France I often wonder why loyal servants get treated like they do, after serving their country. Says he will pop in to see me some time when I told him I would be here a few more weeks yet. Late night drink—cup of hot chocolate and later still my sleeping tablet.

February 13th

5.40 a.m. Trolley about then lights were switched on at 6.00 a.m. Cuppa—7.25 a.m. Breakfast—8.20 a.m.

Been watching cricket from down under—New Zealand. It was the first of the ODI (One Day International) when we lost by four wickets. Later on, after all the necessities are taken care of, physio arrives. Had a walk, then the CPM until lunch break. CC, assortment of cheeses, raw onion and tomato.

13.00 hours—I started a long letter to a pal of mine, then stop when the physio comes in to take me for a walk and the CPM. Had four different nurses, it seemed, looking after me today. It's on the quiet side, so perhaps this is the reason. I bet it will be different tomorrow when the surgeons are getting cracking. Yes, they start quite early sometimes, maybe 7.00 a.m. So the supporting team have to be even earlier than them for all the preparation has to be sorted out with no hold-ups.

February 14th

When the trolley came along at 6.00 a.m. I was reading a magazine called *The Cricketer* which one of my visitors had kindly left me to digest. I have now had permission, whilst lying in bed, to dispense with the brace and only put it on when I am wandering about, so this is an advantage. In fact today is Valentine's Day and those nurses on duty came in and wished me a Happy Valentine's Day, which I reciprocated much to their pleasure.

All the observations completed and what then occurred was very unusual for the staff nurse in charge had left me, whilst I was reading the newspaper, with my feet in soak and then gone for her tea break (had this occurred before you might ask?—could have done!). After I realised that this indeed was what had occurred I worked a towel over with the walking stick which I found invaluable in such times of need—the hand end hooked round the object, then presto it's near enough to grab. Just as I reached successful completion of the task, a sister came in enquiring, 'What are you doing, Percy?' I told her that the staff had been called away. Now there was another change of stockings and both legs been creamed—I didn't mind for I enjoyed this treatment; it made you feel comfortable for my, at times, they didn't half itch! Physio arrives—walk and machine until 11.45 so it left me with only up to the middle page to complete before lunch with *The Cricketer*. I was trying to remember how long ago it was that I had read this super monthly mag—must have been at least twenty years.

Lunch is a toasted cheese sandwich with lettuce and tomato—no sweet.

By the time my walk nurse had arrived!!! Scissors!!! She's a good sport and knows I call her this. I had completed about five hundred words to another pal of mine in Lincolnshire. Hop-stop-hop-stop then the CPM until 17.10 hours. Just keeping around seventy-five degrees.

I added another four hundred words before dinner—and with a stamp am sure it caught the last collection at 18.30 hours.

Another staff nurse had heard that I was back again and called in to see me. She is a truly dedicated one. I would even suggest that her nursing duties came even before family!!! We were talking about her dad who is quite a good age. I told her, 'I bet he is mighty proud of his daughter.' We have a new patient across the room opposite who has haemorrhoids and has had his operation early this morning and is now talking. Unfortunately he seems to think there is not any improvement—so when I had a chance I hopped across and told him quietly that 'Rome wasn't built in a day.' Dinner—roast lamb, veggies and new potatoes. Apple pie.

February 15th

One regular job I have to do is place my teeth back in—yes!!!! top and bottom!!! And of course I like to have them in before the thermometer arrives for a reading (one of the three observations taken regularly during the day) to grip the device in question!! This morning am not sure what occurred but I was way over the top—37+. I realised that an incorrect reading had taken place so I said to the nurse can she try again—after I had given the aforementioned a wash and brush up! Normal reading—35???? Have to check this as am not sure.

All jobs otherwise finished by 10.00 a.m. including a change of clothes which also takes place every day either before or after breakfast—usually after.

Physiotherapist arrives—walk-hop; came back knackered and the walk has not got any longer. CPM until 12.00 hours.

Lunch—jacket potato, grated cheese and pats of butter. I had more enquiries earlier whether I could go on the weighing machine—this was brought to the room after lunch and the staff nurse gave me a reading that made me feel a bit more comfortable!!! Have gained about two pounds!! So I was highly delighted, that's in twenty-three days.

I started and completed a letter to Dickie Bird the umpire whom I had met whilst travelling in New Zealand during January and February 1997. I found him just the same in real life as he portrays himself out on the Square. A no-nonsense sort of chap. I have told him about the problems that I am having and am now letting him know that I have no chance of going to see our boys in New Zealand.

Dinner—piece of boiled fish (plaice), with big helping of mashed potatoes, peas, fruit including an orange.

Mr Mac calls in just after our meal and said that it's time we took another blood sample and also set a date for the next operation. Staff who had been on all day took those notes—they soon put a new dressing on after he had completed his visits. Late-night drink—hot chocolate, watched some telly and later PK and ST.

February 16th

Saturday today, so of course change of waitresses. Early morning cuppa arrives at 7.40 a.m. The waitress has time to have a quick chat! My, it does my eyesight a power of good!!! Ah it does that!! Early morning cuppa, 7.30 a.m. Breakfast at 8.15 a.m. All observations and jobs completed by 9.00 a.m. and waiting for the physio to come along and give me my walkies. A different one, and am pretty sure she had not exercised a hopper like me; she's not sure whether to walk in front or by the side or behind. Yes, of course, I asked her if she had worked with anyone as awkward as me. The reply: 'Well, there is always a first.' Good marks to her. Am sure she had not experienced this sort of patient before but she was pretty smart getting me on the CPM though, as I watched her without interfering with her duties. Anyhow I reached eighty-five degrees without too much discomfort, coming off at 11.45. Lunch—CC, cheeses, tomato and raw onion.

Watched cricket in New Zealand when England lost by 155 runs. Incoming phone call from friends in Gloucester, Dot and Allen, also a couple of Get Well cards.

My, it's getting hard to find space for all the flowers and cards that keep arriving but it's nice to be remembered. Nurse on duty is Pultzer, the collector of flowers that keep finding their way into my room—she must have a heart like a lioness for this sort of kindness seems to spread around; she keeps all the patients in a contented and happy frame of mind.

Rest of day—eating, bed exercises—just moving legs from side to side; hop and walk in the morning and afternoon watched horse racing on the box.

Derrick, my friend called in, pretty shaky but mighty determined. He is the chap being treated for Parkinson's Disease and some days he is quite well and trots in and out with no bother at all but today he just could not get his legs going—that is co-operating with his grey cells or even just to change the position of his legs. This afternoon he is having tremendous difficulty in performing this task.

February 17th

When I had my final wash last night, I managed to knock the towel rail off again, so this was going to be a good start for the day. I told this to the waitress who came in with my early morning cuppa at 7.30 a.m. She caught me reading one of my birthday books—and of course was interested in what I was reading. 'Oh, blooming cricket!' she declared.

8.30 a.m. Breakfast, toilet, wash, shave, change of clothes, back washed and dried—in that order. Reading the newspaper followed, and at 9.45 a.m. physio arrived for hop-walk and CPM. Tony the postman arrived with my mail from home and watched me going through the motions of the machine and saw the vital switchboard move round eventually to eighty degrees—whilst here he also had a cuppa. Maintenance men up to repair towel rail. He said to me, 'What are you up to in this room?' What could I say?—moving around with the brace on my repaired leg. Lunch at 12.00 hours. CC, cheeses, raw onion and a tomato, then I had a dessert. Today—jelly and ice cream.

Afternoon—did some writing, made a few phone calls, then approximately 16.00 hours—a walk with the nurse, then the CPM, a quick last-minute burst up to eighty-seven degrees.

Rest of day—usual checks, observations, eating and generally minding my and other patients (who needed it) affairs.

Mum died 1979 aged ninety-four. This is a first. No fresh flowers on her grave.

February 18th

Most of the staff are moving about taking calls on the buzzer and also observations. 7.30 a.m. early morning cuppa, 8.15 breakfast, all other jobs completed by 9.00 a.m. Then feet up, armchair with a newspaper.

Usually around this time, I have the cleaning ladies come in and do their jobs. Wash, brush-up, hoover, sort out the dead flowers—in fact do anything within reason. One senior staff member of this elite outfit—for some reason, I am always pulling her leg—has been listening to my plans for the bank raid I was plotting. This morning I told her that I was short of a get-away driver!!! And how was she fixed for driving the super-charged vehicle!!! 'Yes, that's all right with me, Perc, but the money's got to be right,' she says, moving her thumb and finger together. The staff nurse came, gave me a walk, then onto the CPM, coming off just before lunch break with a holding achievement of eighty-five degrees—and then I repeated to myself, 'What's the use!!! It's all got to be cut open again—' Soon as I think along those lines, thankfully there is always another incident that is much more important and relevant to the present situation in the corridor or a nearby room. So I can't dwell on this for very long.

12.45 hours doctor came and took some blood, then during this period I had another brainwave!!! Why don't I put some questions and answers together—taking them from the book of knowledge lying on the bed. So this is what I decided to do—find some difficult questions and answers from the book I had received, *One Hundred Lords' Tests,* and send them to my Brains Trust pals around the country. Early afternoon Mr Mac called in to find out the result of blood. Very sorry, not back from the Path Lab—this I might add is quite unusual for all the departments to my knowledge work together, with few hiccups occurring, but I understood that before he had left the other wards some twenty minutes later, the result was with the ward sister who passed this onto me that the blood levels are down considerably and Mr Mac is very pleased.

Several visitors arrived including Lawrence bringing his wife, Debbie along as well—and I must say a very enjoyable afternoon was had by all. Around 17.00 hours I did my hop-step-and stop!!! Then the CPM around eighty-five degrees.

Derrick arrived and was pleased to see he was managing quite well but, according to the head Mrs Mopp, he was a very famous person: this account was witnessed by not only herself but also others. Derrick was trying to cross Palmerston Road when he could neither go forward or go back until some kind people, realising that he was in difficulty, had led him to the other side from the centre of the road where he had been stood stationary with all the downhill one-way traffic honking their horns wondering what all the fuss was about. The police had been called and took him home. He had told me about this episode in his life, just saying he had a job to cross Palmerston Road over the weekend and had to be brought home by the police.

I enjoyed my dinner which was served up as usual piping hot—steak and kidney pie with a nice crispy pastry surrounding, filled with goodies. I did not have a sweet—for what with the three sorts of potatoes, doubt if I could have found space (mash, new, and old!!! Whew!!!).

I had at 21.00 hours a cup of hot chocolate and then just before lights out, pills sleeping and PK.

February 19th

Early morning trolley so I knew who the sister was on duty—the time, 6.00 a.m. Cuppa—7.30 a.m. Breakfast—8.15 a.m. By

9.00 a.m. I had also completed all my early chores: toilet, brace put on (still), wash and back dried as well as shave, change, and rinsed out yesterday's trunks. I wanted to press on because I wanted to complete my questions and answers and get them off to my pals; that's providing that the departmental secretary would oblige by photocopying them. By mid-morning they had been sent and returned, on receipt phoning my thanks.

10.15 a.m. Physiotherapist turns up—then a hop-walk-stop. Am now doing these painstaking steps more each day and am now at least halfway along the corridor. Back on the CPM at 10.30 a.m. Then by 11.30 a.m. I had reached eighty-six degrees, then completed the four letters all with stamps on and, I trust, the right addresses. Again before I closed them all up I checked all the questions and answers, making sure that each one had a complete information sheet; later, one of the waitresses posted them for me—so I would think that they would have caught the last collection. Lunch CC, various cheeses, onion and tomato.

16.00 one of the nurses came in and took me for my walk, then the CPM again. I went upward to eighty-six degrees and kept it there for some ten minutes.

Dinner at 18.15 hours—lamb chop, mint sauce, peas, cabbage, small potatoes with apple strudel and custard. Late night drink—hot chocolate with pills later still at lights out to finish a busy day!! Partly at the office!

February 20th

Trolley on the move at 6.00 a.m. 7.30 a.m. early morning cuppa followed by breakfast at 8.10 a.m., usual jobs then have the male nurse in attendance who is looking after me this morning—not sure what to make of him; the female staff are always getting as good as they give me in the way of lively exchanges but with this nurse I have my doubts if he will respond in the same way—so have decided to leave well alone!!

Reading the newspaper when the physio turns up: 'Ready, Percy?' 'Why, of course,' says I, all ready with my brace firmly fixed into position; to get to point A and back to the armchair is about the same distance and still takes about the same time; this morning it's straight onto bed next and securely tied up to the CPM with a target of eighty-eight degrees. This I reached again without any discomfort. Lunch—jacket potato-grated cheese, two pats of butter and today, I have had a starter which was a fair-sized melon (piece).

Have had a call from the publisher who confirms that I am going to take 500 books when they are ready for delivery. Another call from my good friend, Sue, that she will visit this afternoon—another letter quickly drafted to an accounts department: they have been notified that I am in hospital—so how can you pay accounts whilst you have a stay away from home? My friend duly came at 14.00 hours with my old neighbour, Noreen as her chauffeur, staying for just over an hour—and having spot of tea and a piece of cake!!! My, she is a busy person, bringing me some of her goodies, which included a home-made pot of marmalade.

At 16.00 hours, I received a phone call from David, one of the five recipients of my question-and-answer quiz; he lives in Newport Pagnell, and, as you recall, I only posted it late afternoon yesterday!!! Yes, he received his before he went to work this morning. I said, 'My, that was quick! I didn't expect you to get them for a couple of days at least.' However, he tells me that so far he has not answered any of them for he has not studied them in detail much—but, knowing him, it will not be long before he can answer the majority of them. Also asks me how I am and when would I be coming out? I explained to him that I have to have another operation before I am allowed home and that will not be for a few weeks. Then

Cricket Questions from Lords' Test Matches

1. Famous bowler of the 'fifties who never bowled at Lords (England)?
2. What test match was the only one when none of the Four Opening Partnerships reached double figures?
3. Who, on his first appearance as a Test Captain (England) scored a ton in his Second Innings.
4. (3 Parts) Lowest Test Score (Year) (Country) (Score).
5. Which bowler bowled unchanged in England's Second Innings—with a two-hour break for bad light (clue: the 'fifties)?
6. Which Australian batsman carried his bat at the age of forty-two (still stands today)?
7. 1899: the Essex Bowler W Mead; what was unique about his appearance at Lords when Australia won by 10 wickets?
8. What year did Freddie Truman take his final haul of 5 wickets?
9. In 1935 South Africa beat England by 157 Runs. What did *The Times* blame this defeat on?
10. What year did England play the 200th Test Match with Australia?
11. Sir Don Bradman's knock in 1930 of 254 runs in their total of 729 took how long? 4 hrs 20 min? 5hrs 20 min? 6hrs 10 min? 7 hrs 35 mins? 8hrs 17 min? Or 9hrs 20 min?
12. Which year was the SIX BALL over introduced?

Answers at end of book.

would you Adam and Eve it! A person came into my room and asked me if I was Percy who had run the High Beech Football Club! 'Yes, one of them.' Her reply: 'One of your old footballers, David Bland, my husband, is in Room 153. Well I never! 'My, it's a small world!' I said, enquiring what was wrong with him; when she told me it sounded as if he was here for several days. 'Tell him I'll pop in to see him tomorrow morning.' Next, looking at the clock, it will soon be hot chocolate time.

I have had a busy day again. In the late afternoon. I had been for my hop-walk-stop and lean-been, on the CPM—enjoyed my dinner of roast chicken, cabbage, calabrese and French fries and new potatoes, dessert plum pudding. And best of all, the postman had worked wonders with David's letter—to get to his house in less than fifteen hours.

February 21st

At 5.45 a.m. there was quite a lot of noise in the room next door. I knew an elderly gentleman had arrived last evening—this was my first experience in a hospital of seeing emergency first aid and its importance to our care and welfare. I heard the sister call out quite loudly for him to wake up—then it appeared he was attached to several important wires which connected him to apparatus that every now and again would call out: Check the pulse!!! And more words which I could not quite pick up and only guess at. It seemed a pretty long time but, in actual fact, it was only minutes—of course I had my door open (and I might add very seldom was it closed at any time) and within a half an hour an ambulance arrived to take him off to another hospital. After making inquiries, I was told that he had recovered but the next forty-eight hours would be critical—yes, he is holding his own. What I do know was how proud the nurse was who told me—for she had been one of the team that had fought so hard, preservation of life being the silent thought in everyone's thoughts. As I told her, I was listening to the combined efforts of all those committed, and also willing the patient to make a noise of sorts and praying that a response when it came would be audible to me as well. Unfortunately, this has a sad end for this patient passed away the following day.

9.00 a.m. Took my time going across to see David—he is under the same surgeon as me. He is not allowed to put his foot on the floor; with myself it is the knee that is a problem but, with David, it is his foot—though he is unable to do any work he is pretty cheerful, quickly getting into 'where's so and so?' Considering that I have not seen him for several years, he has hardly put on any weight at all. I reminded him about the time when he was playing in the quarter-final of the Ongar Cup—and he broke his leg just before the half-time whistle. My duty, being the secretary of the club was to try to get some insurance money from the Essex FA for which Tommy Fagg was the county representative. He made sure, by visiting footballers who made claims from the funds, that they were genuine—of course, he remembers all of this but did he remember the figure? 'Five pounds,' I said—and didn't he want to know how much income was coming into the household? Do you remember the year? 'Yes—1964,' nearly forty years ago. The club did eventually get this payment but not for several weeks.

Have you seen '?' '?' '?'. The list was growing, then I told him there might be a get-together in the early part of the summer, but that this was still a hush-hush story and not on the agenda so far, only in the committee discussion. His wife, Carol, was listening all the time to our tales and appearing to enjoy every minute of them.

'Hallo!' Physiotherapist comes in. 'I wondered where you were.' It's time for walkies, so obediently I went and hopped my way to the far-off finishing line just a few doors away—straight onto the bed, harnessed up to the CPM staying until just before lunch break when I had reached eighty-eight degrees. 12.00 hours—CC cheeses and tomato and an onion.

Had a quick nap—for Lawrence had promised to come in after he had done some physio work in Outpatients. He arrives and tells me that he is very slowly improving. His main problem? Will he be able to fulfil his duties out in the middle as an umpire? Obviously he enjoys it immensely. 15.30 hours, next duty—have a trot, stop, lean on the door frame—no improvement on distance; in fact I have almost given up on travelling any distance with all the weight that I have to move around with me!! No, tell a fib, it's not weighty at all—it just feels awkward. Besides, the main task is not to put any weight on the floor—and this I might add is the most difficult job of all. I have to concentrate all the time—to make sure I don't make any mistakes at this stage. I am positive that I must be well over halfway to the next operation—twenty-seven days from my original count of forty-two days, so perhaps less than a fortnight now. I suppose this is wishful thinking for something is bound to go wrong before then: this one per cent is not far away in my thoughts now. Dinner at 18.15 hours—roast pork, three sorts of veggies with new potatoes, rice pudding with a couple of small packs of strawberry jam, (nearly forgot, big helping of apple jelly).

Tried to get another one of my old footballers on the phone—but no joy.

Just before hot chocolate time, David's sister called in to ask how I was and, of course, not having seen her for nearly forty years, I wanted to know how she and various members of family as well as friends were.

February 22nd

It's quiet this morning but the buzzer is going off every couple of minutes—I am not surprised for the rooms are all full up again owing to the operations that took place yesterday. Yes, I have been down that same avenue as well—and know the satisfaction you get when a friendly cheerful nurse puts in an appearance, with a nice greeting like, 'And now what can we do for you?' or 'I shall only be a couple of minutes,' or 'What? Not again? I shall have to get another nurse to help me—be back in a minute.' That's how it was this morning, for there was a nurse short and now they're waiting for an agency one to turn up.

I had my early morning cuppa at 7.30 a.m. with breakfast at 8.15 a.m. Usual jobs in their order and back in the armchair by 9.00 a.m. with newspaper—just starting reading, when David's wife, Carol came in and asked me if I wanted anything. Super; I wanted some Rich Tea biscuits—she was on the way out so she had made an early start and, best of all, I had them before our tea break.

Physio arrived at 10.30 a.m. to take me for my hop-walk-lean-and chat to whoever—and my, now there are plenty of them who I know (most of the staff by name now) and each one telling me how much I am improving; then they are informed that I have to have another operation. The walk continues with the return journey about the same speed—then up on the bed, attached and strapped to the CPM. Press the buttons and then I am in control!!! Just over an hour this morning with degrees at a steady eighty-eight and feeling comfortable. 12.00 hours—toasted cheese sandwich with a raw onion—again I had a starter which was a generous portion of melon.

Received a letter from the publishing lady, then at 13.30 hours, I gave her a tinkle to confirm one or two points in the letter received—those queries sorted out, I then went back into my office to make sure what we had been talking about was correct. I say my office, for this was my wheelie locker beside me, with an open area serving as a drawer, then another side with a locked drawer and underneath a vast area which I had difficulty in managing; my filing system is simply all the papers that arrive are piled on top, so most times I have to ask whoever is passing, whether they could spare a minute—and everyone a treasure, always willing and happy to do so. After each visit, a nice tidy collection would quickly be disturbed again so might last ten minutes. Made a couple of phone calls—also wrote another letter. When the afternoon cuppa arrived I said, 'I'll be glad when I can close the office for the day.'

Physio arrives approximately 16.00 hours for my hop, then the CPM target set for the day was ninety degrees; this I found fine with the wound nicely healed and no sign of any swelling—looks as if whatever target date Mr Mac had in mind might be on. The knee looked fine (from my point of view) for him to work on!!!

My friend Derrick called in just as Mr Mac came—having a look at the dressing which he says, 'Can come off now.' I may also put more weight onto the ground and I can go back onto my Voltarol tablets. Mind you, I had not missed them all that much because I had not done much exercise and the various pills I was already taking were making me forget other body aches. Derrick, like me, had seen the knee uncovered and could not understand that it had got to be opened up again. 'Looks all right to me,' he said. 'That's what I keep saying. It's a good job the heads know what they are doing,' I concluded.

18.00: dinner is liver and bacon with lots of other goodies—have marked up: it looks too good to eat and disturb; how well the chef had presented it for me. My, did I enjoy this!

Later in the evening I rang Sue to find out how she was and give her my progress report—all under control. During the evening I had a visit from David's grandchildren—their ages I can't remember.

February 23rd

Trolley moving at 6.30 a.m. Cuppa at 7.25 a.m. Breakfast at 8.15 a.m. All duties completed by 9.15 a.m. Morning paper had arrived and was studying horse racing form when the physio came in—asked how I was. Told her that nothing much had changed since last weekend; perhaps I was hopping a little further, she seemed to think that I was making good progress as we hopped-stop-and-lean against a door jamb. She then put me on the CPM telling me that ninety degrees was the target this morning.

Three of the weekend cleaning ladies came in to inquire how I was and as I must have been in a chatty mood, I quoted all eight verses of Pam Ayres' 'Poor Dad' without a mistake. I might add this was rewarded with a round of applause—which cheered me up no end. When the physio had taken me for my walk earlier, we had a good chat about what Mr Mac required when he said I could put more weight on the bad leg when putting it on the floor. I must say she was not all that clear about what I was supposed to do. 'Will mention it when I am making up the sheets later but, for now, carry on and be careful you don't overdo it,' she informed me.

Whilst I was sitting there reading the paper, I was also watching the 3rd ODI (one-day international) from New Zealand—England won by 33 runs; the DL (Duncan Lewis) method had to be used owing to restricted overs being played.

Lunch at 12.05 hours. CC, various cheeses, a tomato and a raw onion. Again, I had a starter of a piece of melon.

Afternoon—watched racing on the box, football and the cricket, one-day international again. David Bland went home hopping but Mr Mac is quite happy for him to leave as he is progressing well. He has one of the old-fashioned pairs of crutches to use—and my, can he hop along! I have now his phone number so I can keep in touch with him—sounds as if it's going to be a long job with him.

The lady chef called up to make inquiries about the meal being prepared—again what a person! I told her about the pounds I was putting on, so she said, 'Well, don't blame me.' Dinner at 18.00 hours—a dressed chicken no less, new and old potatoes, peas, calabrese, with rhubarb and custard followed by the cuppa. Late night hot chocolate with a couple of biscuits, then just before lights out—pills.

February 24th

6.00 a.m. the alarm buzzer peals out, so somebody needs help—though quite often I have witnessed that the person who is pulling the cord is not necessarily in a hurry and could have avoided pressing the bell. Usually I found that those who have only been in a few days are the culprits—but they're never ever told about this for their health is paramount in this hospital, regardless of how the staff are situated. This time I overheard the patient saying, 'It's full up (meaning that his bottle was full up and needed emptying). Now could this person have hung on just a quarter of an hour longer whilst all the night staff were working against the clock to complete duties before the day shift started. And talking about clocks, the other night I had an agency nurse come in to do my observations, so she held my hand finding the pulse whilst looking at the clock on the wall to the right of my bed, then she said (foreign nurse—Rumanian?), 'That's fine.' I did not take any notice, only just asking about taking my pulse with the clock on the wall. 'Oh yes I can with that one,' was her reply.

The following morning I said to the day nurse on duty that I had a nurse the night before who instead of using the timepiece on her wrist had used the clock on the wall. 'Couldn't have done.' I said, 'I witnessed this occurrence,' and told her to look at my chart. And there it was: quite clearly a normal reading—as before during the day's observations. Another nurse came into Room 151 wondering why a lot of interest was being shown in the clock on Percy's wall—after an examination of the clock on the aforesaid 151 wall there was a clearly a remarkable difference between this one and most of the others in other rooms (all of them about the size of clocks in school class rooms). This one has a second hand movement going round the same direction as the minute one—mind you, you had to look at it quite closely to observe this action. No doubt, this timepiece could tell some tales, probably in action long before affordable clocks came to be marketed.

After completing all the early duties at 9.30 a.m. the physiotherapist arrived, took me for my hop with the trusty fixed frame, then the CPM up to ninety degrees coming off just before a lunch of roast beef, Yorkshire pud, roast potatoes, Brussels sprouts with dessert apple pie and custard. 14.20 hours—went for a walk then back and on the CPM at 14.30 hours. I was then all ready to take my seat with a good view at the Worthington Cup Final between Blackburn Rovers and my team Spurs, who lost 2:1. Not a bad game and with Blackburn taking their chances, they probably deserved to win. One of the staff sisters who had been on duty, had gone home when finished to watch the outcome; when I saw her the next day, she said all the family supported them and were all shell-shocked at the result.

A good friend of mine who is also a Spurs supporter came

to visit with her husband who is not one. Both stayed for some time whilst I enjoyed my dinner of scampi, chips and peas. I invited them both to have a meal with me but both declined. They told me that the weather was pretty rough. I told them, 'I have been sympathising with whomever has come in to see me. I was told it had been pouring all day and does not look likely to pack up now.'

Cup of hot chocolate later, then about 22.50 hours—the last of my pills.

February 25th

I had already started a letter when the trolley started its journey delivering pills and medicines. It was a bit later this morning for the time is 6.30 a.m. It had been a busy night with the buzzer going off several times—might have been the hours before lights were switched on. Anyhow early morning cuppa at 7.00 a.m. Breakfast at 8.15 a.m. There is a problem with my Flucloxacillin and Ciproxcicin but it is quickly resolved with information received that Magnus (house doctor) is taking blood later on.

In trouble with my wheelie locker—described earlier—where all my papers build up so when I remove one all the others fall out. Fortunately, the nurse is close by to help me out with some kind assistance—this I might add is still continuing. I completed my letter at 10.15 a.m. just as the physio arrived—asking me what progress I had made over the weekend. I told her that I am still to wear the brace but can put more weight on the floor, but I am not clear as to what weight that should be: 'What would you advise?' There was not much forthcoming—as she rightly said, 'I have not been left any directions. We'll just have your usual along the corridor, then wait for Mr McAuliffe to confirm his requests.' Back on the bed strapped to the CPM, press the buttons and then I'm in charge—nice and comfortable, right through to ninety degrees.

Magnus, the doctor came in and took some blood followed by Mrs TT from pharmacy. I have named her after one of the Telly Tubby persons. She is, checking, distributing, writing in the chart and all the time inquiring about this, that, and the whatever—usually with a broad smile that she is always proud to produce on behalf of both of them!! I am pretty sure she cannot make head or tail of me!!! Come to that, does she understand me at all?

12.00 hours. CC, various assorted cheeses, with half an onion and a sliced tomato. After lunch I completed another letter to Peter Walker, the chap who is writing a foreword for my book. It reads very well and am pleased with it as I think, with all this time spent here, it has not in the slightest affected or upset my grey cells. I do know something: when I eventually am released from this hospital, I will design something more straightforward than this locker, which I have cussed again this morning. This does bug me and am sure if these notes are ever taken seriously, this locker, along with all the others, will have a few alterations! If the bed is pumped up, then it's on a level with the top drawer but it's too high to reach the things you require from the lower space. If the bed is in a very low position, this makes it more difficult because you want to get back to a nice neutral placement!!! That's between the devil and the deep blue sea. I still have the drawing in my mind as I type this!!! This will have to wait for another day. I have a hop with the nurse close in attendance after my afternoon cuppa and a piece of cake, always fruit. CPM for an hour—up to ninety degrees. Dinner at 18.15 hours. Piece of plaice, mash, peas, dressed with a slice of lemon. My—it did look nice and I slowly made inroads until finally I had completed everything including the dessert—rhubarb and custard. Lights out at 22.55 hours.

February 26th

Early morning cuppa at 7.30 a.m. All observations out of the way but buzzers are having a good testing this morning. I honestly think that new patients have problems after operations, being sealed up in a room. The cord is pulled to get attention for the tiniest thing. Other older patients, I notice, will fuss about getting their things together the night before, then, through the night, the brain gets really active—more unrest with the buzzer as a form of help and release.

Breakfast 8.15 a.m. Then usual jobs—including nurse giving my back a good examination and the result—I had to hang on to the wall owing to the vigorous rubbing which this particular nurse dealt out. Then my bottom had the thumbs-up—but it's their duty to make sure that the patient is free from bedsores, which I know occurs quite quickly if the patient is lying for too long in certain positions.

Armchair—reading the paper until physiotherapist arrived just before 10.00 a.m. Then followed a debate about the brace. Advice is—use the crutches until Mr Mac offers an opinion. When I have been out hopping—I don't mind telling you—I just wonder how long it will be before my other hip decides to say enough is enough. The right side is the one which is taking most of my weight when I am out on hopping expeditions—so far, touch wood, there has been no sign of any pain and long may it continue. The reason why I am concerned is that I had the left hip replaced in June 1995, Mr Mac told me then, it would not be many years before I would have to have the other side replaced and that is now six years ago.

Back on the bed after a ten-minute walk, then connected to the CPM, staying on for just over an hour with the ninety-two degrees reached.

Lunch at 12.10 hours—toasted cheese, lettuce, tomato, half an onion.

A couple of phone calls after my twenty-minute nap that I had indulged in following my meal!!! Oh dear—what am I playing at? Sleeping at this time of the day!!!

Mr Mac called in and I asked him about crutches-brace-and-weight-on-floor. His reply, with the nurse making notes: 'Yes it's all right to go without the brace now but be careful when you first put your weight on the floor.' I reminded him about the book launch date for April 11th. 'Yes, that will be fine,' also adding that as the blood count was very good, we would soon have to fix a date for the final operation. Rest of the afternoon—cuppa and a piece of fruit cake, a walk with the crutches and no brace or frame, CPM, then 18.00 hours—chicken with chips and peas (leg and wing) then later made a start on two more letters and almost completed them just before hot chocolate time. SP, later PK.

February 27th

Have marked up first thing: 'What a day!!!' For starters, this pen that is today's pen for writing these notes has turned up after it had fallen on the floor, rolled somewhere and then, when the cleaning ladies came round, tried to jam the hoover without success. 7.40 a.m.—night nurse had put all my tablets in a pot ready for taking with my breakfast, observations are done and charted. 7.30 a.m. early morning cuppa. 8.20 a.m. breakfast—senior staff nurse on duty this morning, same one who left my feet in soak—now all long since laid to rest. All jobs finished by 9.15 a.m. Armchair to read the paper—then decided to start and finish a letter to my publisher—that's another person whom I don't know how she puts up with me—am confident that she knows that I have tremendous respect for her and the guidance she is giving me.

Getting carried away for, after completing the first few lines, the physio arrives. 10.15 takes me for my hop-stop-and-lean, progress is still the same as when I started thirty-two days ago, then back in 151, strapped to the CPM for about an hour coming off at 11.45 a.m. Ninety degrees.

The man opposite is one of those patients who has his concerns, problems, life history, diet and umpteen other daily misfortunes all at his fingertips. I received a gala performance in my armchair during four visits from him during the course of the day. Of course, I have met several like this—but I was not even asked why I had been here such a long time. It was only after he had gone to get some history papers to back up some of his tales—and he was not sure of the facts as he had presented them to me—that I mentioned that the knee had got to be operated on again for the fifth time within a few weeks. 'Oh you are not going home yet then?' he remarked. Strange, I have been involved with people from all walks of life, throughout my various careers, and I have found it easy to chat along with anyone. I say to myself, 'There is always tomorrow and maybe it will be my turn to tell him about me.' He was one of many who crossed my threshold during my stay and most had good intentions to improve the person's health and be of good cheer. In this instance I was left to mull over the make-up of human beings.

Lunch at 12.10 hours: the chef has done me proud again. I gazed at all in front of me, not knowing which of the arrangements to start first. Six different cream cracker biscuits—various cheeses, a tomato and half a raw onion. Afternoon, completed a letter, added a stamp and should have caught the 18.00 post, then was popped on the CPM for an hour up to 17.45 hours.

My neighbour across the corridor went home late afternoon, popping in to say cheerio. Sister came in to report that my blood count had come down from over 40 to less than 6. 'It's all looking good, Perc,' she says.

Mr Mac came in stroking his chin—so straightaway I guessed something was in the wind. At once he said, 'The insurance are getting concerned with the situation, so it might be in everyone's interest that you go home for a few weeks, then come back for the final operation.'

And it was only yesterday after my lunch, that he was talking about making a final date for the op. Well I don't mind telling you this was a knockout blow for me, for I felt and told him that if I went home I don't quite know how I could manage as even here with all the help I was getting I still felt a liability at times. 'How much weight can you put on it now,' he asked, 'and how far can you walk?'

'No, I can't put too much weight on the floor.' I'm pretty sure his thoughts were that I should try a bit harder (I have recorded this in my writings) but I realised reading through these notes next day that he was indeed a very busy man. Finishing his conversation with me he said, 'We are, as you know, very busy with operations at the moment.' This was after I had reminded him of the important date that was coming up in my life in April—when my book was going to be launched. Yes I knew like many others, the Holly House Hospital had been very busy since the latter part of the old year—with so many operations coming in from various NHS hospitals, many cases having waited as long as thirty months or more. So after my dinner which was roast chicken, new potatoes, Yorkshire, roast potatoes, cauliflower and dessert plum pudding, I got cracking on a letter to Mr Mac and marked it 'personal', telling him I have recorded in my diary what I said. I should have put down that I don't want to attend in a wheelchair!!! It seems a lot of the nurses are disappointed, but I told them, 'I should think he will have a change of heart for he would not want to send me home if I can't look after myself.' During the rest of the evening, I considered the position I might find myself in and I knew this was going to be pretty awkward at times—well to be truthful, all the time!!! What if I fell over!! I dreaded the thought.

Sister came round at 20.00 hours to say that the physio will tell me what sort of weight I should put on it. She had caught me out of bed and I was doing just that—putting more and more weight onto the affected leg. As I told her, 'It's all right here—all I have to do is press the buzzer and help comes from all directions.' 'Yes that's what worries me, Percy,' she said. I have also noted down how it struck me as odd Mr Mac saying that the blood count was good while at the same time—looking keenly at the knee and it's weird stitching patterns—adding, 'It's healing nicely.' I know I can't see any further at times than my nose—but why say that when he is going to cut it all open again, and start all over again, very shortly. It must be so for he has made sure that it is indeed a temporary joint—that's quite firmly in my head.

February 28th

I am reminded by the night nurse on duty that as I am reasonably agile, it won't hurt me to empty my own bottle, when I asked her; fair enough—a good point and, after all, exercise. I have an early morning cuppa at 7.15 a.m. with my breakfast 8.10 a.m. In the toilet, having a shower—whilst I was attending to this a couple of nurses came into the room to change the linen, calling out, 'Going home today, Perc.' I called back, 'This is news to me.' When I had completed the other jobs attached to getting up, Staff Nurse came in to say the same thing—wanting also to know what time had I in mind for going. I told her exactly the same as the other nurses and Mrs Moppses who also had heard that I was leaving them. Well you can imagine, this was getting to me, because, at this time of day, I had not got a ghost in hell's chance of contacting Mr Mac who was now probably getting prepared for operations. I sat in the armchair reading the newspaper until 9.50 a.m. and, as the physio had not turned up, I decided to ring my insurance company to find out my position—carefully making some notes to make sure that they understood how I felt. A male employee answered the phone—I gave him my name, temporary address, policy number together with the claim number. He told me, 'Wait a minute and I will get your file.' Then after telling him of my position and the difficulties I might find myself in, I got straight to the point: 'All I want to know is—are you going to pull the plug on me?' 'What we will do, Mr Salmon, is I will have a word with my colleagues and then ring you back in about an hour's time, is that all right?' 'Yes, of course, but could you tell me your name?' 'I'm Adam.'

The physiotherapist had now arrived to take me for a walk on crutches, then back in 151 and onto the CPM with her telling me later, when I was taken off, that she is very pleased with me. 11.30 a.m. phone call for me. Insurance company saying, 'This is Adam here, Mr Salmon. First of all, nobody is pulling the plug from under you at this company and you can rest assured of that,' continuing, 'In fact the company is quite happy with the situation. We have had a chat with the hospital. It seems as if no excessive weight is to be allowed to be put on the repaired leg—so it's best to carry on until a final operation date has been agreed. In the meantime, the company and myself wish you well and trust it goes well for the future.' 'Adam,' I said, 'I will certainly recommend you for higher office,' thanking him most kindly. Almost as soon as I put the phone down, one of the porters came along with the wheelchair to take me down to the X-ray Department to have some photos done. This did not take long for I was back with both x-rays before 12.00 hours.

Lunch soon arrived with most of the nurses now informed that Percy was not going home, as one told me: 'You can't go home yet!' Then one of the porters reminds me that the powers that be are sending my election papers c/o Holly House Hospital for a date to be decided. Today, enjoying my cream crackers much more, various cheeses, tomato and half an onion. What a morning! I must say my brain had been in a bit of a turmoil before I had made the phone call, so all I have to do now is wait for a date to be set for the final operation. Have had several visitors during the afternoon and, in between visits, I have completed a couple of letters. As I had run out of stamps, one of the Mrs Moppses, in her tea break, had shopped for me for a new supply. Lawrence came along and joined me in a cuppa and a piece of cake.

One of my last visitors who came in at 17.45 hours stayed for about twenty minutes with his daughter but as he is hard of hearing he did not understand me when I explained to him that the final op was in view. He told me about his ears and how he had come up today to have treatment for them and was very pleased that he could hear so much better!!! 'Yes he certainly knows his stuff—the surgeon who attended to me,' I said and, increasing the volume of my voice, noted, 'I don't think it has made any difference.' 'That's what I think as well,' came his reply.

Dinner—shepherd's pie with veggies and new potatoes, apple and custard for dessert and a pot of tea. Shortly after this when I was settling in to fill in this diary, Mr Mac came in and said, 'It's all pointing to next Friday for your final operation, that will be forty-one days, not far short of the six weeks that we had got you down for originally.' My reply: 'That's fine.' I was pretty excited by this change of plan as you can gather, so I got busy on the phone calling my good friend Sue, to say that I was going to have my final op next Friday and I knew she would be highly delighted. I have also seen a remarkable difference in all the flowers that adorned Room 151. They seemed to have all perked up, with the foliage, dare I say it, 'glowing'. The night sister, when she came in was very pleased that the insurance company was happy and the operation can go ahead in a week's time. Phone calls all done, everyone in the rooms around me is quiet, just the odd buzzer breaking the peaceful surroundings. Somebody had closed my door, must have nodded off. The waitresses on duty with hot drinks are also pleased that I am very shortly to have a final op.

March 1st

I must have had a good night—for long before the trolley had come along at 6.10 a.m. I had completed almost a hundred words of a letter I wanted to get off to catch the morning collection. By 7.40 it was all finished with a stamp on. Breakfast at 8.10 a.m. Then, after I had completed my morning constitutionals, I had my surgical stockings changed, which I might add are changed every day, with legs sometimes being washed, dried and ointment applied. In fact, it has been known to have a different nurse working on separate legs whilst I either sat and admired them or read the racing page! Ah, what bliss!!!! The physiotherapist appears, for she, like a few of the nurses, came in to say how pleased she was that I was stopping to have my final operation done before I go home. I was taken for a walk with the arm crutches without the frame but even then I was finding it awkward to get along and had to stop and recover my exertions caused by just those movements. Then ordered to the CPM for an hour with the target ninety degrees and plus. This achieved at ninety-two degrees.

Lunch at 12.00 hours with the usual CC, various cheeses and a tomato and half an onion. Phone call from the publisher lady who thanked me for my letter—so that was another area where the postman delivered within twenty-four hours—Somerset. A walk with the crutches and a nurse to keep things steady just after an afternoon pot of tea and a piece of fruitcake. Derrick had called in and had the same as myself. Now it's very strange—with a cup of tea you might think with his Parkinson's he would find it difficult to keep his cup of tea steady—yet today it was almost as if his troubles never existed. I remarked to him about this—thinking that there could have been an accident when I invited him to take tea with me. 'No, I feel fine today,' came his reply. Then a walk with the nurse who says, agreed with by other patients, 'You are doing fine.' I don't feel that way—always at the back of my mind is what's going to happen when the final operation takes place and I was thinking like this when I was put on the CPM for my afternoon thrill!!!!!! Derrick might have put this idea into my mind when he said that I might catch another infection. I remember saying to him, 'Gawd forbid.' Anyhow the machine was up to ninety-two degrees and I was feeling reasonable with no pain anywhere—so am quietly confident that the bug which has plagued me has been laid to rest.

Dinner—scampi, new potatoes, cabbage, peas with dessert apple pie and custard. Noted that I took a few incoming calls!! I don't think in my lifetime, I have ever, and I know it's true, ever spent so much time on the phone—all through my years, I have not spent so much of my time answering the telephone or for that matter sending calls out to friends and relations!! 'Oh well,' I said, 'hang the cost. There are a lot of people concerned with my welfare and health—and those people are very important to me.' I have made a small note in my diary—don't forget to mention the phone and the account that's building to the credit controller.

March 2nd

Up at 6.30 a.m. Started a letter to a good friend of mine who lives in Theydon Bois who knows I am in hospital but I have not been in touch with her by letter, only the phone—I know a phone is all right, yet it seems awkward at times when conversation goes searching for words, and this can apply to both parties on the phone. Anyhow I can quickly put together sufficient words to make a half-decent letter—and I know when she opens this one that she will be pleased as punch. 7.30 a.m. early morning cuppa with a biscuit, then 8.20 a.m. breakfast—nothing changes with regards to my breakfast—two poached eggs on two buttered pieces of toast, then baked beans on the weekend to help the staff. Showered, everything under control and completed by 9.00 a.m.

When the physio arrived to take me for a walk, another chap came in to see me—now we do go back a long time for we were both in the ATC (1065 Squadron) together—dare I say it—nearly fifty years ago and after spending all this time round Loughton, he has decided to move up to Norfolk to be near his son and family. I ask him: can he do me a favour, not important for a couple of weeks or so—just when convenient? 'Yes of course, Perc.' All I want him to do is make some photocopies of some digital snaps that one of the patients took whilst here.

Lunch at 12.00 hours. CC, various cheeses with tomato and onion—it appeared that the waitress's tea trolley was late as the waitress staff were light on personnel but it never fails to turn up. This lunch-time, it was about twenty minutes before you could hear it making its way along the corridor.

Had another walk by myself later in the afternoon and then another one after dinner—which had been a nice fish and chip one with a few peas, with the pot of tea not far behind. I have not been on the CPM—it does not seem to have made any difference for I am now doing exercises on the bed and off it. What a blessing the donkey pole is—for I quite fancy myself at swinging up from floor level (carpet) and plonking myself just where I want to be—without too much further movement.

For the last few nights, I have had a lady pop in to have a chat—she has had a knee replacement, and seems to be doing fine; tells me that she might be going home tomorrow. 'You don't want to worry,' I said, 'they will not send you home if you are not capable of looking after yourself.'

March 3rd

The night nurse is on the move at 6.00 a.m. armed with tablets for me and others—mine in a pot. I was half asleep at the time and, after examining mine, noticed that the Flucloxacillin was missing. This was quickly put right and was taken with my others at breakfast. There is a minor panic again this Sunday morning for the waitresses are short-staffed—and with thirty patients (I am told) in and only two staff, they surely needed help, especially as one had a shocking cold which she told me she had had all week. Breakfast though was not far behind its usual time of 8.00 a.m.

Shower—followed by all the regulars including the change of DVT stockings with also a wash, leg massage and a creamed application by the nurse on duty. My, she did take a time with them both!! Yes of course I enjoy this—I would be telling a fib if I said I didn't!!

Back in the armchair reading the newspaper, when my friend the postman arrived with three of his many grandchildren—I must say that the oldest, a girl, made sure that her brothers were behaving like perfect little gents, always quick to stop being naughty, when told by their elder sister. I bet she is going to be a school teacher—could be wrong!!! As soon as he left, the physiotherapist appeared, walked me along the corridor; then CPM until the lunch break—roast lamb, potatoes, peas plus mint sauce. I also had a starter of a piece of melon, but am being good, and have started refusing the sweets, always on the menu if wanted. I wonder how long it will be before I can refuse the apple pie—must try a bit harder!!!

One of the Mrs Moppses came in with some photographs which had been left at the office for me. The flower lady came in to see me—am pretty sure this is the first time I have met her—but she's another very busy person, I understand, for her duties are to water flowers in pots and vases, leave the plants looking fresh after she has tidied them up. There is not much doubt that all my flowers looked more healthy after she had seen to them. While she was in the 151, she told me her daughter, one of the waitresses, had told her about me—I said to her, 'I'm sorry; I am getting a reputation, but it's none of my doing,' continuing, 'Everyone, as far as I am concerned is super and they all know because I tell them all.'

Derrick called in and is pretty steady—but I know he is glad to reach the armchair to sit down and recover; his first remark is to ask what has the big chief got to say—this is regular each time he visits. Today I tell him that I have not seen Mr Mac today so far—which seemed to satisfy him. After he has departed, I then went for a walk towards the business end of the Cedar Ward—The Bridge End (so called for this area is where all the comings and goings start from—decisions made, taken, delivered, errands started, stopped, checked, double-checked). At times, the doors to this area are so busy with doing all this that it is incredible how it ticks over so efficiently—reaching this area I decided to return to 151. On the way back I called in to see a patient who had been here for nigh-on two weeks. She had a different type of CPM machine that was providing the passive movements just as well as the one that I was using. Stayed for a chat—which helped to pass the time away. I went on my CPM when I got back to room 151, reaching around about ninety-two to ninety-five degrees. Evening meal—scampi, chips and peas with a melon starter. Watched television this evening for a time, until my hot chocolate arrived just before lights out, plus my late tablets delivered by the night nurse. There was also a result from Melbourne, Australia concerning motor racing—Michael Schumacher had won again.

March 4th

Night staff nurse at 6.30 a.m. coming round to do observations—but I had already started on some correspondence, this to my friends in East Sussex who were kind enough to send me a get-well card now and again, so I thought that I would get cracking to get a letter in the post to them today. Early morning cuppa with breakfast at 8.15 hours. Then general duties all finished by 9.10—which included a shower and also a change of stockings by the staff nurse on duty—who told me that nurses were short this morning. Even then, in no time after I came out from my hideaway, the linen had been changed with telephone, buzzer, glasses, pen, daily paper lying neatly on the bed!! Can't be bad!!! I always asked under my breath—the last day I am in Holly House Hospital and ready for going home, who I would like to give a special hug to!!!! At 10.00 a.m. decided to go for a walk. I see one of the boss lady physios: 'Are you safe enough?' She knows full well that permission had been given for me to tread the boards!!! Had a quick chat to Peggy, asking her how her knee replacement was progressing. 'Very pleased,' she said.

Back in 151, physio put me on CPM which I stayed on until lunch arrived. Without bothering the nurse I managed to slip out of the harness and enjoyed my meal without the aid of the buzzer: CC, various cheeses with tomato and half an onion—no starter.

Magnus, the resident doctor came in and took some blood ready for Mr Mac's attention when he got back from Paris. He had only been gone twenty minutes, when Mr Mac himself came in, looked at the wound and said, 'It looks good.' I spoke to him about our rugby team which had lost 20 points to 15 points saying, 'Our tactics were all wrong.' To this he answered, 'I couldn't agree more.'

During the afternoon one of the nurses (who again is one I want to give a big hug to when I leave this establishment) is concerned about a patient further along who has eaten something which has upset her. Passing my door with her finger and thumb holding her highly sensitive nose, she wasn't the only nurse doing this! In fact, I delayed my exercises (walking ones) for I was leaning out of my open window for some of this time. Then all of a sudden, one of the Mrs Moppses arrived with two canisters of a fragrant aerosol which not only alleviated the atmosphere but interrupted all the joviality which was unfortunately connected. This only works for a while, for very quickly it started up again!! The same thing has occurred down in Room 135. The all-clear is relayed, windows still open; I'm sure this particular day was one I shall remember for a very long time with all the stops and starts, concerns, unease, uncertainty, the buzzer on the go. Made the Monday afternoon cuppa and slice of cake a bit different. The dinner came along a bit later than normal at 18.30 hours. I know there had been quite a lot of serious concern for the patients absorbing this pollution, which had crept, for some reason, right down to the captain's bridge, if you please!!! Anyhow—there are lots of reasons why the meals are behind schedule at times. I think we are very fortunate to have the waitresses arrive so promptly, especially today. Of course, every one of them is saucy, cheeky, friendly, good humoured and quick-witted, arriving at 151 with an en-bloc chorus of, 'All clear, Perc.' I enjoyed the chicken with all the veggies in attendance, plus the rhubarb and custard!!! I did not even consider any complications that might arise from eating the dessert. Late night chocolate arrived also a bit later, in fact at 21.10 hours. I had enjoyed the television for there had been a programme on about Admiral Lord Nelson. Lights out at 22.00 hours.

March 5th

6.30 a.m. Night staff nurse came in to do my observations plus my tablets. 7.15 a.m. early morning cuppa and 8.00 a.m. breakfast—with all my other duties beckoning me, I did not delay in going to have my shower, or doing all the other jobs. What I did notice was that after I had dried all over, my legs had a withered sort of look about them when I looked at them. It must be to do with the DVT stockings that I was constantly wearing day and night. So when another nurse put in an appearance after I had rung the buzzer (to confirm that all my jobs had been completed), she looked at both legs and said, 'I'll get some cream straightaway for them. You will have to have them done more regularly.' At 10.00 a.m. physiotherapist appears and takes me for a walk. Have now trebled my distance from a fortnight ago, then back on the machine—she seemed happy that the target was ninety-two degrees. 'As long as it has reached ninety degrees, that's the knee nice and free now,' she said.

For lunch today, the chef had made us a fish pie; this was a meal in itself but the new small potatoes that came along with it! How could I send them back plus the Brussels?

I was soon restless again and like anyone else—what next to do? Mind you, I did not have many options—and, thankfully, Pat Potter, an old pal, came and stayed with me for a good one and a half hours, refreshing our memories of early days at Sappys, the local builder who employed us both. It was then walking time and, for this exercise, I had a male nurse as my companion, then I was strapped to the CPM for about an hour. This was convenient for the telephone, when it rang for I only had to reach over and pick it up. It was my pal from Somerset informing me how the cricketers were shaping up—without us two, we who could only sit and watch the coming series of three test matches against New Zealand on television. Still it was nice to hear from him. He told me that he was not making much headway with the quiz questions that I had set him. 'Were they difficult?' I asked him. 'Difficult! Those questions are suitable for professional contestants and I am not in that league,' he replied. He asked me if I had heard from our other pals, three of whom had gone out to New Zealand to cheer our boys on in the ODI and a couple of tests. 'No, not yet, but I am sure there is a letter in the post from Martin or a postcard,' I said.

The same nurse took me off just before dinner and also said he would bring my tablets, which, as I have mentioned before, I like to take with my meals. I had eaten my scampi, chips and peas together with a large helping of sponge pudding and custard when the nurse turned up with my tablets. Of course, he had a perfectly logical excuse and, though he's only been working here a few weeks, he had quickly grasped, like the patients had, that five minutes, or even a couple does not necessarily mean that.

I had come to realise that on the way to wherever to run an errand for a patient, another errand gets remembered or maybe another duty crops up—perhaps help is required to assist a patient in dire need. The original errand is slowly, but never completely, pushed further and further back until I feel sure the brain clears and resends the message. This workload throughout the day seems to give their grey cells few worries, despite the heavy burden it places on them to remember this and that. And, of course, I only see a very small percentage of what goes on during the twenty-four hours when several shift changes mean new staff must take over responsibility for the patients' needs.

Hot chocolate at 20.45 hours with my last tablets including my sleeping tablets: Temazepan—I think that's the correct spelling; lights out soon afterwards.

March 6th

I have finally completed letters I started a couple of days ago and am now down to my last one—these had stamps on soon after the early morning cuppa arrived at 7.30 a.m. Breakfast at 8.15 a.m. Shower—with all general duties accomplished by 9.15 a.m. Both my legs are much better and the same nurse is on duty—wondering if they ought to be done again. But I was not on her list of charges so she told me that she was on tomorrow and would be looking after me then. 'Oh all right then,' I said, 'I'll wait until tomorrow.' You can see what this pampering was doing to me. I can honestly say never in my whole life have I been treated like I am when I am a recovering patient. I have made a little note about this, thinking, 'What am I saying, how much longer am I going to stop here, being looked after and treated like royalty?' I have still got to have the final operation which now is only two days away. As I see it I could be here another three weeks!! No, surely not!!!

Today I had not had my regular paper, the *Daily Express*, so another one of the Mrs Moppses, who delivers them went back and changed it specially for me. I know I said to her at the time, 'I will recommend you for higher office!!' This pet phrase is one that I am using more and more often. The paper situation resolved, I had a quick read of sport page and looked at crossword. Exercises!!! The physio had told me that as long as the nurse was nearby I could walk, so this was next on the list. Coming back, I called in to see a chap named Ted, who had come from Whipps Cross Hospital into Holly House Hospital to have his prostate problems sorted out. He told me that he had been waiting for three years and now is also having to have a new knee fitted whilst he was here as a patient. When I told him how long I had been here, he exclaimed, 'Cor blimey, mate, I am hoping I shall be out of here by the end of next week.'

Then as soon as I got back into Room 151, and I don't feel quite so bad as when I first started out (knackered), the physio appeared to put me on the CPM machine, where I stopped until lunch!! Whew, the lady chef who is in charge today with meals has done me proud again. For it's a crime to interfere with any of any of the display in front of my eyes. If there had been a note to say don't touch I would have fully understood and would have borrowed my neighbour's camera and photographed it first before cutting into this creation. I would like to say I ate the lot but partway through I knew it was going to beat me. So I kept selecting only the choicest pieces. Still I did well tackling two-thirds of my meal. During the time I was eating my lunch, I noticed that a gardener was cutting the grass outside my window down below and every now and again a whiff of new-mown pastures would waft up, giving me a lot of delight.

I had forty winks afterwards and just an hour and a half after my first sniff of grass-mowings for the year I was on a walk, then the CPM for roughly an hour. It was while I was just relaxing I received three separate phone calls including one from a friend of mine, who told me that her son had got a mention in *The Times* about his nuptials taking place in a few months' time. Another call was from another old cricketer and umpire. So the letters posted a couple of days ago had reached East Sussex, as he said, 'Received it yesterday morning.' The post can't be too bad then, whatever people say about deliveries up and down the country.

Dinner at 18.20 hours. This time a fairly large piece of plaice, chips, peas and several slices of lemon. I was asked if I wanted some rhubarb and custard as there was a spare one being offered. I politely turned this down. A walk followed; called in on Ted, asking him how he had enjoyed his meal. 'Like a five-star hotel here, Perc, isn't it? Might change my mind about going home the end of next week.' Hot chocolate, tablets and lights out in that order followed.

March 7th

Today I had decided to put together a letter to the director of nursing at Holly House Hospital; I think nearly everyone had heard about the loss of her dad. Remember on February 21st I noted down in my diary that a life had been saved in the next room to me. Duty sister staff and myself were overjoyed that all their efforts had been worthwhile. Unfortunately, it was not to be for, as I have recorded earlier, he passed away shortly after being admitted to another nearby hospital. So I thought that I would send a letter of condolence to her, which I could get typed perhaps by one of the typists working in one of the offices on the next level up. I know this would give her immense satisfaction for I'm confident she would appreciate a few kind words of sympathy for and on behalf of all her many friends here at Holly House Hospital.

Room 151
Holly House Hospital.
07 March 2002

Dear Jill,

It is with much sadness that I am writing to you, trusting that the passing of your dear dad is more bearable and that everything went well yesterday.

As you know, I only met him just the once when I was hopping past his room and looking up saw that Ernest was my neighbour. I said, 'Hello Ernest, I'm Percy and I live next door.' 'Don't call me Ernest, I'm known as Norman, pop in any time,' was the reply.

I was unprepared for the next morning's events when Sister and her team worked like Trojans and the pleasure it gave us all, not realising that their success was only going to be temporary.

What I do know Jill, is that Norman must have been mighty proud of you and your commitment to your profession and I am sure that in putting these few words together I am speaking not only for myself but also for patients and staff alike with whom you have day-to-day involvement.

I, like many others have been down the same road you are now travelling on; the pain will be there for a long time but knowing how you 'travel' into wards and rooms after a visit, if your personality has not made that person improve during that brief stay, I do feel sorry for them. 'With laughter', 'a smile'—the best medicine.

At this sorrowful time, our thoughts are with you and your family.

Respectfully,

Percy Salmon
PS I think 'buzz' would be a more appropriate word after your visits!

There were a few words that I was doubtful about as regards spelling and am sure she would correct them. So soon after I had completed all my duties I left the newspaper, and got stuck into the letter—a draft form soon took shape. When I reread it, it looked pretty decent to me. It was then delivered up to the lady in question via another one of the staff who was on my chocolate pay roll. Knowing how efficient this typist was, I guessed she would sort this out during the day. The physiotherapist appeared to see how I was getting on, also to take me for a walk, then back to the CPM. Whilst I was on the machine, Lawrence came in after his visit to the Outpatients' physio, telling me that things are improving slowly with his hip replacement but, as they told him, it is going to be a long job. 'Umpiring?' I asked him. 'Oh yes, this year should be all right,' came his reply. I was still on the CPM when my letter came back, all nicely typed out—with very few alterations to the original script. On the internal phone, I straightaway rang her to thank her for her kindness. The ninety-two degrees target was comfortable when the physio arrived to unstrap me, and she was pleased with my progress.

Lunch at 12.30 hours: CC, various cheeses with tomato and half an onion with a pot of tea within twenty minutes.

I had a quick nap, then a walk along the corridor to see a new chap who had his leg in plaster when I passed yesterday. His name was Dave and he plays golf. He told me that he plays at The West Essex Golf Club. I told him I had been associated with that course from a very early age. He was telling me that he was going to have a new hip. I don't suppose this is very strange but it's surprising how many golfers come in and have those hip operations.

Back in 151 I had already seen the sister in charge about one of her nurses who says she can cut my hair and had kindly offered to give me a trim in the nearby toilet facilities, providing that it did not interfere with her duties. That's fine.

It had been worrying me for days that I was going down to theatre tomorrow and of course I wanted to look respectable for this. It did not take long for Scissors (the name I gave her straightaway) to perform this duty. I was sitting in a chair with just a small looking glass in front of me and could not see what cutting was going on, only her movements behind and over the top of my head. On completion, another mirror was found for me to approve and I must say that I could find no fault with it. Straightaway, a half-dozen nurses appeared from nowhere, each admiring Scissors' work and of course I gave her an extra big hug.

A walk along the corridor then back on the CPM with the machine holding steady at ninety-two degrees, for I had an inkling that this might be the last for some time.

Dinner—fried plaice, chips and peas. Pot of tea, no dessert, with, at 22.45 hours, a cup of hot chocolate and later at 22.45, my usual tablets. I summarised my day, with how many nurses had come in just to see my haircut. I daresay it made me look quite different, for as I had worked it out it had been seven weeks since my last one and normally I go for less than four. All agreed that this particular nurse had made a splendid job of Percy's haircut.

March 8th

An old chap of ninety-four has been brought in during the night and is in quite a lot of pain from the fractured leg he is suffering from. One time when the sister answered his buzzer, he seemed more than a little confused. I heard the sister say to him, 'It should be better now that you have had your operation.' 'Have I had my operation?' 'Yes.' His reply, I am informed: 'Now can I have some more of my medicine?'

During the morning I found out what this medicine was, for it was a lovely rich amber colour which no doubt was doing him the world of good.

Nil by mouth after 6.45 a.m. So all I had for breakfast was two pieces of toast and an orange juice. Did not do much the whole of the morning, only read the newspaper. Nearer my appointed time of 13.45 hours I had visits from Mr Dodd, the anaesthetist, followed very quickly by Mr Mac, who had brought a form with him for me to sign. Shaking both their hands I wished them well. With Mr Mac saying that, 'Everything points to being successful this time,' I remember looking at the portrait on the ceiling prior to the theatre but did not have much chance to study it, for I was soon sent to sleep. Looking at the clock in the recovery room it said 18.10 hours. Then back in Room 151 (the action room) at 18.30 hours—all wired up and connected to a monitoring machine. As soon as I was placed on the bed, it was noticed that the drainpipe for the rubbishy stuff clearing from my system had been tucked away beside me, coming up from theatre, so this jar was collecting muck and unloading it straight into the bed. This was quickly sorted out with clean sheets, top and bottom, and a rubber underlay directly over the mattress to avoid any problems that might arise in future. It was not long before I was allowed a cuppa but did not fancy anything to eat, though I was offered a piece of toast. I had a nurse constantly in attendance. During the many hours they seemed to sit with me, either talking or reading—and this is true—you find out a lot about a person who is prepared to negotiate your every whim, within reason. I had a male nurse looking after me through the night, who I must say could have picked me up with one hand and thrown me through the window. Yes, a giant of a man with huge hands, but he knew his stuff for when the night sister came in after a call for help had been answered by her, to help change the sheets again (and yes a second time as well), she made it quite clear to me that I was in good hands. Each one started talking to each other in medical and technical terms and both understood what was occurring with the monitoring machine standing like a silent sentinel beside my bed, with an occasional blip or two. What a marvellous machine this is. Temperature, heart, blood pressure, blood count—it's charting everything on a chart which includes times any changes are being chronicled to my body. Whew! Both my gowns have also had to be changed plus the dressings covering my new permanent prosthesis. In his country of origin—Nigeria—he has got a large family and, as I gathered right away, the church plays a big part in his life.

March 9th

I had some drinking water for starters, then later on, at 7.05 a.m., I had a cuppa—then at 8.15 a.m. I had my usual breakfast, eating everything that had been placed in front of me. Then got a phone call from Sue, who wanted to know how I was progressing. I told her I was all wired up with the monitoring machine approving of all what's happening to my body and recording it on a graph. 'Percy, as I've told you before, it's a wonderful machine, isn't it? I'll pop in as soon as you feel better. I'll leave it for a day or two until you have got rid of a few of those wires.'

I have not done much all morning, just read the newspaper and listened to the bleeps of the monitor. I had my cuppa and biscuits at 10.20 a.m. Mr Mac popped in to see me, saying, 'We shall have to let the wound heal first, before we allow the slightest movement. It's most important since, in the first instance, a blood clot became infected.' When he mentioned this, I noted it down straightaway, for this was the first time that I had been told how the infection had come about. For some reason this made me feel a more contented person and think that I must make sure that I wear those DVT stockings for as long as it's necessary.

Lunch—ham, eggs, chips, peas; dessert—apple strudel with custard. Ate the lot, I have noted down. Afternoon, I was glad I wasn't my old self for I know I do chatter and there were several visitors including pals way back from school days with their families. Then finally when I thought that all the pots of tea had been warmly welcomed and drunk, another visitor in the shape of my vicar, Jonathon—well, from the old parish where I had spent seventy years and the majority of them pleasant ones. In fact, one of my pals, whom I had not seen for some thirty years said to me, 'Blimey, Perc, I thought they was going to cart you straight from the post office to the churchyard.' My reply: 'So did I!' Those last remarks we made to each other, shortly before Jonathon arrived. It's a mighty strange world, isn't it (our vicar) turning up within five minutes of mentioning his churchyard? Whilst he was with me he said, 'Would you like me to say a prayer for you?' My reply: 'Yes, if you think that might help.' I thanked him in due course.

Dinner at 18.00 hours—mouth-watering time again. Lamb casserole, new and old potatoes, carrots; then rice pudding with two sachets of blackcurrant jam. I have also marked down a melon for starter. Hot chocolate later.

March 10th

Had a reasonable night but had to have a change of sheets during the night, owing to them being bloodied. This is because of a tiny leak where the stitches are. Will have to pray more now I have had a visit from our vicar.

Had an early morning cuppa at 7.30 a.m. and, as this is Mothering Sunday, I am surprised that I have got a cuppa so early, then again taken aback that the tea trolley delivering the breakfasts was prompt at 8.10 a.m. Again, I ate all my breakfast, two poached eggs, extra helping of baked beans with a couple of slices of toast and marmalade with a pot of tea. Then it suddenly hit me. I had to remember when I had last gone to the toilet! Yes, that was the day of my operation, now over two days ago. So at 9.00 a.m. I asked the male nurse on duty if I could have a bedpan. I don't mind telling you this is a struggle for not only do you have to try to support yourself on one leg but also use a bottle at the same time. After several minutes, when the sweat had started to stain the top sheet, I gave up, pressed the buzzer to let the nurse know that mission was not accomplished. 'You will have to have some Milpar,' were his instructions to me. The sheets changed at 9.30 a.m. I am glad that I was not still in the throes of the mission that failed for my pal, the postman Tony, had arrived with the post but could not stay long, but long enough for him to have a cuppa and a biscuit with me. My friend Derrick arrived and he wanted a cuppa as well; no problem as there was no possibility of getting stuck into any exercises. I was severely handicapped this time, with no prospect of even going on the machine in the near future. Before long, while reading the paper, I had another visitor from High Beech: Roxy, a person who was recovering from an operation herself, and quite jubilant—the vicar told her that I was a patient here as well, when he was visiting her yesterday. She is very much involved with horses and seems a very caring person all round. I asked her how Jan was; this was my name for her daughter who was born on January 1st!!! When this happy event occurred, I told her (Roxy) that to my knowledge this was the very first New Year baby that I had witnessed or knew of, even going back to when our family first moved here—when my great grandfather helped to build the first chapel and very first place of worship. It was called St Paul's and was in Church Road, built in the 1830s. 'She is getting on famously now, Percy,' she told me, knowing straightaway to whom I was referring, continuing, 'She is helping out in our new place, working as a waitress.'

I almost forgot one of the most important occurrences of today, for I had made a special page for this because it seemed at the time to be rather unique. My early morning cuppa had arrived via one of the younger waitresses who saw me wired up and grabbed my hand, asking if I had had a good night. It was then that the monitor, which was registering a steady ninety-seven degrees went berserk. The needle registering all my movements had decided to operate differently with another person's hand now firmly holding mine!! I said, 'It's you holding my hand, you have rapidly changed my body temperature!' 'Can't be!' she replied, gripping even more tightly. It was when the needle started to go completely bananas that I managed to free my hand and as soon as I did so the needle gradually came back to its original position. If I hadn't witnessed it I would have said somebody is pulling legs; not so! I defy anyone when your hand is being gripped by a young waitress who would turn anyone's head, to maintain the same pulse rate, temp, blood, etc. Of course, she was full of this—how she had played tricks with the machine in 151 and whenever she put in an appearance for the weekend duties, we would have a good laugh as to how she had almost silenced my monitor. Of course, I had to name her the mystic monitor maiden, the MMM.

Lunch arrived—CC, various cheeses, a tomato and half an onion.

The afternoon I have seen my friend Chris, the veterinary surgeon, who I must add straightaway is a super person. She refers to parts of my body as if one of her larger animals (horse). This I can quite easily follow if it's explained to me by her; very similar problems arise with both the horse and human frames; then, of course, malfunctioning of limbs followed by tender loving care to get the patient back to normal with appropriate treatments. She stayed for some time telling me that once the monitoring unit was happy with the way my body was receiving the various drugs and all the graphs were pointing in one direction I would start to improve more quickly.

I have noticed before that when a visitor arrives, an important duty will be postponed. In this case the sister in charge (as soon as my friend had gone) came in with her scissors and cut off all the dressings, and cleaned it all up, saying, 'That looks fine.' There was just the one place towards the bottom where it appeared to be still weeping a little; it seemed quite open before another smaller dressing went on. Dismayed later, for Spurs had gone down in the quarter-final of the FA Cup, losing 4-0 to Chelsea.

Dinner—chicken and roast potatoes, carrots with dessert rhubarb and custard. I had a choice of several desserts but decided to select rhubarb for it might start things moving for me—for since early morning, it had been worrying me that to keep on eating like this is not doing me any good at all. I have also noticed that the drain plug that is taking all the rubbish away from my knee, which has been changed regularly, is now appearing to have more waste coming down since sister cut the dressing off. At the time, I did think perhaps that the dressing might have been a bit tight around where the pipe starts from and then thought, I'd better not mention this in case I might have been right.

Hot chocolate time, and the monitor is playing up, for the male nurse, who'd just come on duty had to come in on two occasions to sort the buzzer out because it keeps firing off on its own. Then at 23.00 hours, he taped it up so all was well before lights out. It had been suggested by the night nurse that as it is now three days since I have been to the loo, I must take some Milpar; this is a laxative which will guarantee me some action—'Perhaps before you have your early morning cuppa.' 'I do hope so,' I said.

March 11th

6.45 a.m. I had my observations done followed at 7.30 a.m. by the early morning cuppa with a quick look outside at the weather—cloudy conditions. Flowers inside all look perky. What a morning! I have marked this in my diary—so you may depend that the norm was not the case today.

I felt I wanted the bedpan almost from first light, even when the robin outside had started singing. At 7.30 a.m. early morning cuppa, then breakfast. Ate all that had arrived and enjoyed it. There is another male nurse on duty this morning. Very quickly, I called his attention as he was passing by the door telling him I would like the pan please. This duly arrived (low and streamlined). This I quickly found out made it very difficult to use for it kept sinking into the mattress, and, what with using the bottle at the same time, which made it even more difficult. The nurse came in and seeing that I was getting nowhere fast said, 'Do you need a taller pan?' This quickly arrived—what an improvement! I was now perched up on the bed like a sailor sitting on top of a Conning Tower on a submarine. I put extra efforts into this and—magic!! At last I felt great relief and looked for the buzzer which was nowhere to be seen. I daresay it had fallen on the floor (this proved to be correct). It seemed ages before another nurse came along and I could call out that I needed help. This was quickly attended to, my posterior also creamed and a nice tidy-up in general bestowed on me. Of course, we all had some good laughs and still do about this unhappy episode, when I hadn't opened my bowels for some three days and more. In fact, heaps of suggestions have come forward in the course of time. One that even makes me smile and grin now as I am typing this down!! 'Why didn't you sway from side to side??!!!' I ask you— perched up on top of the bed and hanging onto the donkey pole for extra leverage and support. I do know something— I don't want to be in that position very often.

It was not long after this and when I had just found my newspaper, that I received a visit from the terrible twins, staff nurses, they did not know I referred to them with this nickname—both were always ready to pull someone's leg. Of course, I was in a right state to be plucked, with barely any defences. Fortunately, the phone rang. It was my good friend Sue, wondering what sort of night I had had. It was at this moment that both staff nurses started with first of all, 'Stop it, Percy,' then all sorts of tiny screams, giggles, laughs, stifled shouts, etc. Sue, at the other end of the line was saying, 'What on earth is going on in your room, Percy?' There's me trying to stop the staff from mucking about! 'I daresay you know what's going on, Sue, for this is two staff nurses come in to check me over; it's all under control.' It was back to normality within a few minutes with all the linen changed and the bed made respectable again, dressing changed, back washed and wiped very vigorously. Talk about getting a patient better. These nurses had been around a long time and knew how to make sure a patient was cheered up. Don't think I was the only one getting this treatment. Far from it—you noticed, with pairs working together, that happiness and frivolity went hand in hand and worked wonders on every room they had on their daily list. Change of stockings as well. Excitement over for one morning—you might say—far from it.

Mr Mac came in, wants to look at wound—so the dressing comes off. It's still weeping blood in two or three places, but he says, 'It's looking good,' and, quite pleased, tells me, 'You can stand, walk and load bear, but don't do too much.' Roxy came in to say cheerio for she was very much improved, only stayed a couple of minutes, telling me I had got a reputation with a lot of the staff. 'What me! In my state of health!' I almost shouted at her.

Another staff nurse came in to change the dressing recently disturbed, and also took out the drainpipe which had only collected very few millilitres. In fact, through the night it had not added any more, so its removal enabled me to have more freedom with the repaired leg. A visit from the physio, no doubt on the instructions of Mr Mac, telling me that I can get out of bed: strictly no bending, then use the frame (without wheels) to the door and back. Time—11.25 a.m. I can name other mornings like this here, but this is in the top ten!!! So far!!!

As the lunch is late today (I was not to know this) I had started a letter and almost completed it to my publisher lady by the time I heard those wagon wheels on their way at 12.30 hours. Scampi, chips, peas, with rhubarb and custard for my dessert.

I have now heard that the old chap next door has come

from another local hospital and a nip or two of the hard stuff is his favourite tipple. The nurses think the world of him, for he seems to get visitors all day long (mind you, I had my share this morning) but I am told he is quite deaf, so that's the reason why his music is turned up often. As soon as I get moving I shall certainly pop in and make myself known to him. Mind you, I don't think that we will have much in common, for evidently he has been involved with politics all his long life.

The afternoon started with a message to say that the person from 153 who had diarrhoea problems is going home today. Several canisters of fragrant perfumes have evidently been used but there is still an unusual flavour in that particular room when an extra deep breath is taken for those with sensitive noses. It's nearly 14.00 hours and John, the chap across the corridor who had his prosthesis done the day before me, has come across to find out a bit more about the noise coming from this room this morning. I quickly told him about all the goings and comings. He said, 'Yes, I get the same treatment.' I said, 'Looks as if you are making good progress?' 'Yes, going for a walk along the corridor now'—looking out enviously to see him disappearing. A few minutes later, another good Samaritan, Noreen arrives with her companion Sue, this time bringing a few of her camellias from her garden; they stayed for over an hour—both very caring people especially visiting the likes of myself. Sue had brought me a pot of her jam. I told them, and they could see for themselves, how the girls were looking after me with the flowers that have been arranged around me in 151. It was not long after they had left at 15.20 hours that Derrick arrived, staying for a good hour and a half.

Evening meal—a bit behind tonight, for it was 18.30 hours when the dinner trolley started its chatter along the corridor. Chicken—roast, new potatoes, carrots; a starter of a piece of melon.

Made a couple of phone calls, then my last visitor for the day—Mick Fairfax, from a family long associated with High Beech, telling me his mum is back in Whipps and is not too good. 'You are in the best place here today, Percy, for it's been pouring with rain all day.' Hot chocolate later when he had gone and, later still, just before lights out—my tablets.

March 12th

6.45 a.m. I started and completed a letter to the librarian at Loughton (about the publication of my book); he is also a very expert fuchsia grower and exhibitor. 7.30 early morning cuppa—8.10 breakfast arrives. Roxy, who I thought had gone home yesterday, has had another night with us. At 8.45 a.m. I asked for the bedpan. Nothing like as inconvenient as yesterday but nonetheless it was certainly a struggle to resolve my immediate urgency—with less straining and oh dears! A successful ending came approximately ten minutes later and within another ten minutes, I had been made presentable again, all the regular duties sorted out and the bedlinen changed; DVT stockings put on by the nurse looking after me. Then time to pick up the paper—alas, no glasses! At one time there were five people in 151 but to no avail, the locker, toilet, my carrier bags—everything had been searched, not once but several times. Mrs TT arrives, goes into the toilet, comes out with my spectacles in their case—peace again. Among those searching were the waitresses, cleaning ladies, nurses, both male and female. The physiotherapist came in, had a walk along the corridor with me for only a short distance, just taking short steps, still no bending. Could well be because the skin is so fragile, where it has been opened and stitched up five times; any excessive pressure will start it opening again.

Cyril, my neighbour evidently has another name—Alf—so it seems that agreement has been reached that it is the former that is to be used.

Lunch arrives at 12.10 hours. Salmon, calabrese, three fair-sized new potatoes. I did have a sweet but cannot make out what it was—I know there was a nice juicy apple which I peeled, ate and thoroughly enjoyed.

Afternoon—among my visitors, Tony, a friend from High Beech, his pal John, motorcycle Dave, Pat the post, then later still, Derrick. All had a good stay with a cup of tea as well as extras. I put together another letter to Sue, thanking her for her visit and an incoming surprise letter from another old footballer, Snowy, which I kept reading over and over again, it was so funny. Dinner at usual time, consisting of CC, various cheeses, tomato and half an onion. Later after hot chocolate time, I had two doses of Milpar. Nurse telling me if this does not sort you out, we will have to give you double amount.

March 13th

6.15 a.m. The sister with her trolley is on the move so all her nurses are buzzing about as well. Observations, tidying up, even changing sheets but fortunately mine are okay. I asked one of them about the situation of the brace. Could one of them give me a hand to put it on, then I might be able to go to the toilet myself? Not on your nelly—or words to that effect. You will have to use the pan if you want to but wait for the physio to come in, then they will let you know. So I suffered in silence. Cuppa at 7.30 a.m. with breakfast at 8.15 a.m.

There was a real buzz about the wards this morning for before I had completed my toast, the day nurses were on parade already. Had been making beds in other rooms—so it was quickly my turn. I asked the senior one about the brace—if I could put it on I could go to the toilet myself. 'No way. If Mr Mac says no brace, then that's what he means. We have to follow the book,' she continued. 'Wait until the physio comes in, then ask her.' Later when the guvnor of the physios arrives, I explain the situation to her as I felt if I could sit on the raising piece am sure I would be more comfortable than squatting on the bed. 'Yes that will be all right providing you keep it straight with the brace on.' Then the other physiotherapist comes in, took me for a walk with the fixed frame looking after me. Straightaway I said, 'I think I can use the toilet now—more food, cups of teas and etceteras.' Sat on the throne for some twenty minutes with very little success after usual-push-shove-strain-grunt and lots of oh dears. Back on the bed with help from the nurse plus the donkey pole— what a godsend this is for now I have it off to a fine art: I grip it with one hand, then swing the whole of my repaired leg up and over the bed, keeping the whole thing straight without the slightest hint of sag anywhere. I have also had another change of sheets whilst I have been away along with another vase of flowers, so I know which nurse is on duty.

Put a couple of letters together, one for accounts here, who keep sending them to my home address; it gets sorted eventually—like this morning. It was during this time I was out with my pen and paper that we had an almighty blast of wind that blew the window open and sent most of the plant life on the windowsill onto the floor, plus the Get Well cards. One of the nurses heard me call for help as she was passing by, came in, closed the offending window, then not only put everything back to normal for me but also put papers that I could not reach into the lower shelf in the locker. I then had one of the male nurses come in who had told me earlier that he was looking after me for his spell. I generally get my tummy jab around 12.00 hours and this time I was glad when he had completed this task. If he could understand me—am not sure—but he certainly understood when I went 'Ouch'! This, it seems, is something either you have the knack of or you haven't. Ninety per cent seem to stick the needle in without you 'ouching' but the other ten per cent—be prepared!! I generally say to that percentage: 'I had to do the same when I was learning my trade—make mistakes on the big learning road, but be prepared to listen.'

Lunch at 12.30 hours. CC, various cheeses, tomato, half an onion.

Having forty winks just before starting another letter—one of the staff sisters came in and I told her about the difficulties I was having with my bowels. 'I'll mark you down for some senna, that will sort you out, Percy. I will have to get the doctor to write out an order for you.'

I got stuck into a letter to my old pal in Somerset—inside a graphic account of a story, Snowy my old footballer, had worded to me in his letter to me yesterday. I will reveal all later in this script. I also filled him in with progress with my book.

Racing from Cheltenham: I am glad that there is not a bookie who visits, for he would have taken some money off me this afternoon—it was some exciting racing though.

Derrick called in at 17.00 hours and seems very steady today. Like he says, he has good days and bad ones. Am sure he gets a great kick out of these visits for, without a doubt, it is correct when I call it action room. Hardly ten minutes goes past without something either inside or outside occurring. This sort of activity certainly keeps the conversation flowing. He stayed until the tea trolley started its route along the corridor from the lift. I had scampi again with peas and chips; no dessert but my tablets are taken with my food. Another nurse on afternoons and evenings took me for a walk. A visit from Mr Mac soon followed—when he helped to undo the dressing. He took a good look and said, 'It looks all right. You can stand on it a bit longer, walk a bit further and sit out in the armchair. Yes, of course, use the toilet but keep your brace and leg straight though.' He added, 'In all probability you will be able to go on the CPM machine on Friday.'

It's also been mentioned that dressings like steri-strips or similar can be used. Two nurses were with him and both making notes; I'll have to wait and see what's used. He looked worn out—for he had just completed a busy afternoon and evening at Outpatients. I said to him, 'Have you had a busy day?' Looking at me intently he said, 'Sometimes, I think the clinic is just as difficult as the theatre.' 'But it's not very often that you get awkward old devils like me—one per-centers,' I said. He just smiled and left 151 to visit another patient opposite. Hot chocolate arrived with the night staff attending to my dressing later, then tablets followed by lights out.

March 14th

I had been told to use the brace if I wanted to when off to the toilet. So at 7.00 a.m. I paid my first visit unaided. Leaning on walls for any support I felt necessary, I managed this quite comfortably and didn't worry as a nurse was not far away changing the soiled sheets. I have marked down 'Much better', after my visit.

I had had an early cuppa, also breakfast at the usual time 8.10 a.m. Keeping my brace on, I found, seemed to be an improvement whilst lying on the bed, because when it is off I do tend to wriggle about, doing twist and turns. The physiotherapist arrived and took me for a walk, without the brace, furthest that I have been so far—right to the end of the corridor, almost to the bridge.

Lawrence had arrived and stayed for a couple of hours. He had not been with me for long when I had to have the dressing changed because the blood had started weeping through. I just could not believe it because I was more than confident that the infection or whatever had cleared up. I had made steady progress from my operation last Friday and then looking forward to using the CPM machine tomorrow—Friday. I could have cried. I buzzed for the staff nurse, who like me, was surprised that it had started oozing like it was. She very quickly put on a fresh dressing. Time now 10.45 a.m. By 11.30 a.m. I had to buzz her again for it had all wept through again. At 12.00 hours—pill and injection. Staff telling me that Mr Mac had been informed and, though pretty busy, would call in around about 13.00 hours. This in no way stopped me eating and enjoying my lunch—a fine arrangement of CC, various cheeses, a tomato and half an onion. Mr Mac had problems of his own in theatre, so he did not call in until much later in the day. In the meantime the staff nurse who was also the unfortunate staff (senior) nurse on duty as on Christmas Day said to me, 'What have I done, Perc, to deserve this?' I told her, 'I feel the same way. Why pick on me? I have always paid my bills, taxes, never owed anyone anything and can look any person straight in the eye. Why me?'

We both had a good laugh, but only I could continue mine for the poor staff were busy with patients backwards and forwards to theatre. They had two porters to help, who, like the nurses, knew me quite well by now. At 14.25 I had an agency nurse come in, after I had pressed the buzzer, to see the blood weeping from the dressing. She went out and called the senior sister, who came in and said, 'What have we been up to now, Percy?' I replied, 'I'm blowed if I know.' She had me tidied up in no time. Yes of course it had to be a pressure bandage. You can gather how I was feeling, for now I was almost frightened to move a muscle in my repaired leg, scared that the slightest movement might start it all off again. Sure thing, at just before 16.00 hours, the agency nurse was passing by. I called her because I was sure that the blood had oozed through again. She removed the dressing and, lo and behold, it was nothing like as bad, with just a little blood coming from the area where one of the metal stitches looked as if it had not connected properly. Of course she did not agree, but made a good job with the dressing. It was while this agency nurse was in 151 and talking to me that I realised what might have caused the blood to start. I mentioned to her that I had been doing some leg exercises—quads contractions. I was sure it would have been this that set it off again.

I rang Lawrence and told him what I thought might have started the blood to flow because he had been in 151 when it all started. 'Yes, I bet you're right, Perc,' was his reply. I could recall quite clearly after he had reminded me that the problem began when I first started to lift my leg up and down.

Dinner at 18.00 hours—a piece of plaice with all the trimmings including pieces of lemon—no dessert.

Pills have arrived, not at the specified times but give or take twenty minutes. This, as you can gather, was one of those days which I am pleased to say do not come round too often. At 19.20 hours, Sister called in, had a look at wound and changed dressing, telling me that most of the wound is healing nicely except for this one place. Mr Mac has been programmed about my condition and has told us that we have to cut out the injections and wear another DVT stocking which includes the Ciproxcicin. I said to the sister (senior), 'If my bad luck continues, do you think I could change the room? It might mean a change of good fortune.' 'Of course we will, Percy.' This might be the start, getting rid of some more blood—again this might be strange but this is the very same senior sister who was on duty on Xmas Day, as well. Would you Adam and Eve it? Have almost completed my notes for today except that I have not marked down any hot chocolate. This I must mention; there was hardly a night went past that one of the many faithful waitresses didn't bring me in my cup, a smile, a laugh and a turn of foot.

March 15th

Early morning trolley moving along, have not noted the time but I know who the sister is and her second lieutenant, who I ask if it's all right to go to the loo. This I did as I have the walking frame; the dressing over the wound was dry and remained so while I paid my visit. Early morning cuppa arrived at 7.30 a.m. followed at 8.25 a.m. by breakfast. At 8.50 a.m.—out to toilet and wash. All jobs completed, clean linen, back washed, dried by a nurse who has a worried look about her this morning. I might be a bit inquisitive later. The physio arrives and takes me for a walk without the brace, just a dressing and the frame and there and back without any leaking. Have had a swab taken this morning, which goes to path lab for analysis. 12.30 hours—lunch arrives. CC, various cheeses, tomato and half an onion. Have also had some washing done for me which also includes the DVT stockings that did not take long to dry, for in that toilet at times, the temperature gets beyond a joke.

But who am I to complain while I am being so luxuriously looked after with many extras? The nurse who is looking after me until her changeover would like to change my stockings, sort my legs out and give them a cream. This was enjoyed by both parties especially when I was asked if there was any more washing that needed to be done, as well as the dirty DVT stockings that were removed earlier. 'Yes, of course,' quickly finding some more in the locker. 'Have you had your back done today yet, Perc?' I was then asked—of course I had. Then followed a white lie. One of quite a number I would say! 'No, do you want to give it a going-over for me?' A few minutes later the back felt like new again.

The next task was when the physiotherapist said I could go for a longer walk if I felt like it when she arrived. So I went a bit further this time, going right round to the end of the L-shaped wards. This, with various stops, took me some twenty minutes as this direction took me past the action area or the bridge. Very seldom have I seen this particular T-shaped area quiet—human traffic of all denominations arriving, delivering, collecting keys, unclipped, clipped again to belts, doctors and surgeons, administrative personnel, Mrs Moppses', visitors inquiring about loved ones, visitors leaving, patients doing likewise from early morning until late at night. This command post hardly has time to breathe. A time machine with questions and answers always at the ready, open day and night continuously for twenty-four hours. Back at 151 after I had enjoyed talking to several new patients on my excursion; most seemed to be coming in for minor operations and only stopping for a day or maybe two. Watching cricket the rest of the afternoon, England versus New Zealand.

Dinner at 18.15 hours. Lamb chops, calabrese new potatoes, carrots, mint sauce. Mr Mac called in at 19.30 hours, telling me that it's important that we do not do any bending at all. 'If it comes to the situation that you are unable to bend it at all, later I will bring you back into Holly House Hospital for a day, send you to sleep and put you on a manipulation machine which will bend your knee automatically.' He could see me wincing. I said, 'It sounds painful.' 'No,' he said, shaking his head, 'we must let it heal first before we do anything.' Removing the dressing, the staff nurse finds that it is dry and that the blood has stopped. Must have been a reason for my observations were not done until after I had had my hot chocolate.

Saturday, March 16th

6.45—a letter I must get off to Mrs Farquher—or Peggy, another dear friend of my old mum. I know that she is aware that I am in Holly House Hospital but have not let her know what sort of progress I have been making. Only just one phone call. I daresay when she receives this, when it's completed, she will want to pay a visit. By the time that morning cuppa had arrived at 7.30 a.m. I had finished this one, some three hundred words. I had started another one to Pat and 'Ante' and by 8.00 a.m. the diary as well. Breakfast, then the toilet to begin my daily regular duties. Magic, back to normal—makes me feel good for it's surprising, this is always at the back of my mind whenever I am tucking into something. Where's it all going to if there's no movement down below?

'Paper here, Perc,' one of the Mrs Moppses called out (her regular duty). A nurse came in to give my back a wash and wipe over. This nurse, one of the old school, no mucking about, good solid wipe all over, finishing with a comb through my hair.

Physio arrives with orders that—nothing is to be done, no exercises at all with just a short walk along the corridor, toilet is all right but no further without assistance. I said, 'Surely I can walk along the corridor—if I can walk a short way?' 'No, that's my orders.'

12.30 hours: lunch arrives—ham, eggs and chips with the Flucloxacillin tablet arriving just as I was beginning to think that I had better make a start, for it seemed such a shame to disturb anything in this attractive repast.

Senior nurse came in and took dressing off and replaced

this with a clean one. While it was off, I had a good look at it. There was very little blood; the place where it is leaking is right near where I had noticed the metal stitch—which does not look as if it's fixed properly. Watched the telly all the afternoon with England beating New Zealand by 98 runs, having set the New Zealanders 550 runs to win; they were all out for 451 with Nathan Astle scoring 200 runs off 153 balls and last man out—final score—222.

Evening meal at 18.20 hours, just a light meal. I had CC and various cheeses with a pot of tea soon following. 20.00 hours—nurse came in after I rang the buzzer to report that the wound was leaking onto the lower sheet. I generally put some tissues down to help the situation, which I had done this time. After a fresh dressing had been applied I said I hope that's the last one for the day. 21.45 hours—night nurse came in with tablets, observations all done with a count of 160/88. This staff nurse on duty is a smart person, very big built and legs like tree trunks (it appears) and I must say with a personality to match. 12.20 hours: lunch—roast pork, roast potatoes, vegs, cab, no dessert.

I was thinking about a little nod, when a nurse comes in: change of stockings with a wash and cream and, as there is also a slight weeping of blood, it's decided to change the dressing—apply another pressure one, which hopefully would be the last for the day. Thankfully, it was. I am pleased with the knee for it has always been quite hot compared with the other one but for some reason, they were both (it seemed to me) at equal temperatures. At 16.00 hours, I turned the telly on to watch football. It was then that I had a visit from Lisa, Margaret's granddaughter. Margaret, from the next room, had told me earlier in the day that she would send Lisa in to see me, and 'you will find her pretty talkative'. 'Yes of course,' I said. She told me she was aged nine. We had a good old chat but unfortunately Lisa said hardly a word!!! But she was an avid listener, because I told her all about my birthday and the choruses of Happy Birthday I had enjoyed at various times during the day.

Derrick arrived just after Lisa went, so we both watched Arsenal beat Aston Villa 2:1 staying until the dinner arrived at 18.10 hours. Scampi, chips, peas with a half of melon for starters.

I have a male nurse looking after me—am not clear if he is supposed to be looking after me from when his duties started at 14.00 hours. However, I am not too pleased with how he does his injections (an agency nurse who to me does not have the same gifts that our own register of nurses has—well, that's my opinion). There are several jobs he has watched me do, while he is either taking an avid interest in my blue book, or telling me about his previous hospital where he is employed for most of the time.

I rang Patrick, the agent who is looking after my book, to find out if we are going to meet the launch date appointments. He, like me, doubts if this will be met, for several unforeseen elements are arising, so we wish each other good luck. I tell him that I should be home the next weekend starting the 22nd. Hot chocolate later with tablets followed by lights out at 22.00 hours.

March 17th

I must have had a good night for by 7.25 a.m. this same staff nurse had completed all the observations, then said to me, 'I will pop and get your tablets,' well before the early morning cuppa arrived. While she had been away, I had looked in the bed—blood. When she reappears it's no problem and very quickly sorted out; finally a pressure bandage had been applied with a change of sheets all recorded in my little blue book inside fifteen minutes. While she was doing these important tasks for me, she asked, 'Did you manage to hold your tent down? Don't you remember me coming in as you were having a rare old dream, also holding your hand.' 'You're joking!' I exclaimed, adding, 'So it was real what I was dreaming about, and my tent.' Within an instant of her mentioning the tent, it all came back to me so I told her all about the dream and its real-life source.

I was together with several other children camped out in a field called Alderhills; this was a higher piece of ground overlooking Aldersgrove Estate, I could not have been very old for my sister Winnie was there, who was four years older than me. This was quite clear for we were both in Taffy Davies's gang, a school bully, who was in charge of operations and who no doubt had detailed me to help to put the tent up. It was my duty to drive the pegs in. Staff nurse said, 'It was quite distinct and clear what I heard: "My tent is trying to blow away." I must have only been seven or eight at the time; staff says to me, 'Would you have slept in them all night?' My reply: 'Not likely, it was too far from home.' She asked, 'Do you remember holding my hand?' I truthfully said, 'I am not clear about that, sorry I can't be more specific.' I must say I was very impressed with her for her attitude oozed confidence and for a big girl she seemed to glide around doing her duties with very little hassle.

Early morning cuppa brought by one of the younger waitresses, another one who each time she came into the room—oodles of confidence with a nice cheerful smile: 'And how are you today, Perc?' Of course, I said, 'Much better for seeing you.'

Breakfast at 8.30 a.m. Then followed all regular duties also a change of stockings, then the Mrs Weekend Moppses arrived with the cheerfulness continuing—bright, breezy, chatty and full of beans; exactly the same as the weekday ladies, asking as usual, 'Anything you want, Perc?' 'Not to worry,' is the usual response when any of the nurses are called out when the buzzer sounds.

7.00 a.m. Observations all looked after by the male nurse (Jack Johnson look-alike). I know he is a jolly fine nurse with excellent credentials as I have mentioned but he gives me the creeps. It's just how he moves about quietly and stealthily; my imagination runs riot when I think of him, not knowing that he was behind me as he tapped me on the shoulder and me turning round to follow his frame onwards and upwards, to me it's frightening. I am glad that as far as I know he is the only nurse built like this. I also know through the grapevine here that he is a very dedicated and devoted parent. I had also formed this opinion when we first met, whilst he was looking after me when I was recovering from my final operation. What I do know is that he has only been with us a short while as an agency nurse. It is now fifty-three days plus two since my arrival.

March 18th: Day Fifty-three plus two

I had to have a very early call out by pressing the buzzer—time—1.45 a.m. The bed was having more of my blood—am sure it's because I wriggle about. The night nurse on duty quickly changed the sheets, applying another pressure bandage. I have also marked up Day Fifty-one plus two. Observations at 6.30 a.m. Early morning cuppa at 7.30 a.m. By this time, as you have realised I am wide awake early, so this morning is no exception when I heard the medicine trolley start its rounds, I started writing a couple of letters, both addresses strangely in Pyrles Lane, the road where I live. Breakfast at 8.15 a.m.

then all vital jobs accomplished within half an hour of me clearing my plate; jobs included a bit of washing.

Another male nurse is on duty and looking after me for the next few hours. I am sure he will make a good nurse but it's no good him thinking he can earn a bonus by the speed he moves about and rightly I have told him so—am not sure if he can understand me, but most times he seems to take it in. However, his movements do not slow down. This morning he had started to change the sheets and knowing he had come straight from another patient who he was looking after, I asked him politely if he had washed his hands. 'Yes,' was his reply. I then said, 'Well, I would like you to wash them again.' He went straight to the toilet, making a noise as if he was singing and reappeared with a big beaming smile.

Lawrence, the umpire arrived at 11.30, to say he is visiting Outpatients and will call in later to see me and have a chat. When he did eventually come back after I had completed my CC, cheeses and half an onion, I was busy completing my letters. Mr Mac also visited me at 13.00, and the nurse removed the dressing. Unfortunately, it was weeping blood. Mr Mac says, 'It's looking good.' Poor old Lawrence: I could see that he did not think it was looking good by the look he gave me—I have noted down: 'It's a bloody shame,' a pet phrase which I have been using now for some time. One of the physio ladies has also remarked when this is occurring, 'Bloody bleeder!'

When Mr Mac had departed, I explained to Lawrence, 'What he really meant was that the whole of the stitched area was looking good!'

The male nurse was still on duty when he was asked to put the fresh dressing on along with the pressure bandage. I felt this was going to be difficult for him—all due respect, but I don't think he understood, so I told him that I wanted the senior staff nurse to come and put it on. She came straightaway.

She instructed him (the male nurse) on the importance of the bandage. This same nurse is on duty through the afternoon as well so when Lawrence decides to go, I ask him if he (Lawrence) can give me a hand with the brace. This task is difficult to do. It's just fixing the Velcro straps tight and in the right place at top and bottom of leg. It is important for the brace to be put on correctly for if it's not aligned properly it's awkward to move about and painful near my ankle. Helping me, he hardly said a word. I told him a couple of times, 'No, not like that.' I know I should not be doing this, but I like to think I am being helpful.

14.15 hours and right next is a note that I must check on. It says: 'Now into my 58th day. I'll have to check on that for I know headquarters and my own records should tally. I have also marked down that I feel pretty cross about this situation and am sure all this time with only four walls is getting to me. If only the blood will stop oozing.

14.30 hours. Keith my cousin gives me a tinkle, telling me that it's been pouring with rain where he is working. I told him that's exactly what it is doing here. It's not left off all day; he asks me how things are going. I tell him that I feel all right in myself, if it would only stop weeping blood—hardly stopped since my operation back on the 8th.

15.15 hours—pot of tea arrives with a piece of fruitcake, then exercises along the corridor. This time a nurse takes me as far as the bridge and back. By this time another nurse has joined us, both deciding that as my stockings have not been changed today they ought to be. They agreed to take a leg each, washed and dried, cream applied. There was a slight dispute over the putting on and position of the stockings. Of course as it was my leg and I was the one who was wearing same, I would have to be the sole judge of this. So I told the one who had worked on the repaired and stitched leg that she would have to come second as there were more obstacles than the other: 'Tomorrow—if you want the same job and you have the time to spare, you can change legs over.' All agreed and passed unanimously. Again I reminded them that each is doing a grand job and I loved them all. Have also noted, 'If only bloody thing will heal, I could soon be out.' Dinner at 18.15 hours—roast pork and potatoes, veggies, Brussels. No dessert. Hot chocolate—20.45 hours with lights out at 23.00 hours.

March 19th

6.30 a.m. Observations all done and dusted. 7.20 a.m. early morning cuppa. Had also started and completed two letters before breakfast arrived at 8.15 a.m. Wash, shave, all tasks undertaken successfully. Also the regular change of shorts and washing accomplished. Back on the armchair, nurse comes in and says, 'What's that blood, Perc?'

'Oh no!' I said; sure thing, it was oozing again. So by 9.25 a.m. I had also had another pressure bandage applied.

One of the maintenance men has arrived to fix up my dimmer switch. Certainly he has brought all the necessary spares but as it's an electric switch from a bygone period, it will only work if the whole thing is replaced by removing the whole box, so of course this took longer than anticipated.

At 11.45 a.m. the physio has been in to say that I must not do any more walking until wound is healed. I wonder how long that will be?

I have enjoyed my CC, various cheeses, tomato and half an onion as well as Cyril's music in the next room 153!!! Mind you, at times in the last few days, it has been trying different patients' patience when he winds it up and this afternoon was not going to be an exception. I first had a phone call from the agent, Patrick; as Patrick seems concerned about the book launch, it seems quite likely that we shall have to postpone it until 25th April—for there are more snags arising, and for my own sake too. Every time I talk about the book and consider dates, I imagine doing a book launch and my very first signing carted there in a wheelchair—I always shudder at the thought.

Cyril had by this time repeatedly re-played the Royal Air Force March Past. I have been told he is a stubborn old ****!!! I don't mind telling you I was looking forward to meeting him as the nurses tell me he is such an intelligent old chap, with very positive faculties, and all of them think the world of him. I am beginning to change my mind, for now it's really getting to me. Since he has been in 153, there have been loud and brief slices of opera music. Before lunch, and now into the afternoon, the nurses and the cleaning ladies repeatedly try to get him to tone it down but it has not the slightest effect! As soon as he's by himself, he winds it up much to the nearby neighbours' displeasure. Colonel Bogie! Can you picture that? I am then informed that he is supposed to wear his hearing aid but when he takes it out, he can't find where he has put it, so a lightning broadside starts with, I'm sure, the walls vibrating with those drums and cymbals. I phone the lady in charge of household duties. Tells me that it's not her department. 'Sorry, Perc, but it's only the nurses who can deal with that situation.' Then one of the senior staff nurses came along the corridor, went into Cyril's room, and when she came out, peace had been restored, with all parties satisfied with the outcome. Cyril was more content as the bottle(!) was now close by again. At last, nurses and other staff were able to converse with each other again.

Most all the staff including the waitresses are all having a good chortle about the racket that has been coming from Cyril's room. Time was now 14.35 hours. It was later on that I was informed that he had the Big C and that it had reached an incurable situation. I don't mind telling you, I felt terrible about this. If I had known that Cyril's stay here was going to be of short duration I would somehow have covered up my ears to help to nullify the sound. I was more determined than ever to see him, though it was now going to be mighty difficult as physio has said, 'No walking until it's healed.'

Later on Derrick called in. I told him that earlier we had had some loud music being played next door and he would have enjoyed it immensely, for we had the RAF band playing Colonel Bogie, not once but three or four times (being an old RAF chap) until he was told to turn it down. Both of us had a good laugh as I was moving my walking stick about, like Cyril was doing, in time with the band. He then stayed long enough to be envious of what I was having for my dinner—shepherd's pie with all the goodies. Later I made a couple of phone calls and then came a surprise visitor, one of the earliest motorcyclists I have witnessed in my lifetime. He was just eligible to ride, when I saw him on a Triumph many moons ago. I stopped on my own motorbike and said to him, 'You are not old enough to ride that bike.' An instant reply: 'I was sixteen yesterday.' It is Mrs Farquher's son Michael, who told me his mum had fallen over and is now heaps better and sends her love.

Hot chocolate with tablets, dressing seems to be okay. It might be better if I did not move much at all. Lights out just before 23.00 hours.

March 20th

Early call out at 4.00 a.m. I had noticed blood on the sheet where I had moved about during the night. Sister soon came in: old dressing replaced with new one—change of sheets, top and bottom. Ten minutes: of course I always say I'm sorry.

Early morning cuppa 7.35 a.m. That's unusual. I want to go to the toilet, so I had to take great care how I used the frame to get me there and back.

8.20 a.m. Breakfast then all my usuals. The nurse Scissors looking after me is the hairdresser who I am sure is eyeing my hair up for future business and I know that it needs it too. Back washed, dried, also change of stockings.

Back in the armchair with all necessities close to hand and reading the paper, when the phone rings. My pal Pat had found the bookshop in Epping where the book launch is to take place, giving me the number (of course I am excited). For Lorna, when I got through to her tells me, 'Yes, *Breakout at Sixty-five* is out next month—25th, and will have plenty of stock.' I have another phone call from another old pal, Derrick who lives in Harlow (not many of us original reformed members of the High Beech Football and Cricket Clubs left); can he pop in to see me this afternoon after lunch? I managed to pop in and see Cyril and wish him well. His daughter was with him. He thought I was his new nurse. I also noticed his 'medicine' bottle was half empty.

12.10 hours: CC, various cheeses, tomato and half an onion. A phone call from Win, another person who is still in shock after losing her husband Horace, a good pal of mine. Wondering when I will be coming home? 'I can't say,' I tell her, 'not until the wound heals.' I must say it's nice to find, when you are indisposed as I am, how this phone keeps you looking forward to it ringing. A large parcel arrives from the printers!!! A copy of the book (no less!!!!!) asking me to do a final read before the presses start to roll—it looks magnificent. Of course I have enquiries as to what the parcel is, three nurses and three Mrs Moppses. I must mention here straightaway that there is only one person who knows anything about me becoming an author and my book *Breakout at Sixty-five* and that's Mr Mac who was sworn to secrecy months ago.

Derrick, from Harlow arrives and of course we get back to the good old days, him staying for nearly an hour. Along the way, he tells me about his two sons, one living in the USA, and a granddad to boot. Rest of the afternoon until dinner, I read through eighty pages and can find very few mistakes. I have also to confirm with the printer that I have received the parcel in good condition. This quickly completed, the chap Lyn, tells me that as soon as I am released from hospital, then he will get the books sent to me: 'Shouldn't be any more hold-ups now,' but now I have recognised that One Per Cent is a figure not to be laughed at any more.

Dinner—chicken, calabrese, carrots with new potatoes; had an apple. Hot chocolate, with tablets later—this still includes my Temazepan SP.

March 21st

I started reading at 5.30 a.m. Correcting the odd one or two mistakes that I thought should be changed before the final press of the switch.

I am also pleased to say that the wound has held up—the dressing looks good. Early cuppa at 7.25 a.m. Breakfast at 8.15 a.m. All other duties performed and managing to move around very gently, sat in the armchair. Then another male nurse who is looking after me this morning says, 'There is some blood leaking from your dressing,' so while he was gone to collect new materials, I reprimanded myself, but for the life of me don't know how I have managed to open it up again. I had really crept around from A to B, B to C also in the toilet I had been very careful—remembering that I had had to bend it very slightly when I sat on the raising piece on the pan.

Holly House Hospital operation day today and already it seems as if it's going to be a busy day. Lawrence, the umpire arrives, then another chap named Steve comes in from across the corridor; he has also had a Kimberley hip fitted like Lawrence. It was quite interesting to hear how one had made progress while the other knows what he has to face in the next few weeks; it's going to be a long haul—with, like me, lots of patience.

Physio arrives and tells me I can go for a walk but not very far, so orders must have been changed.

I completed reading my book just before the lunch break: toasted cheese with a bowl of lettuce salad.

As I had found one or two quite noticeable mistakes during the course of reading *Breakout at Sixty-five* straight after dinner, I tried to ring the publisher, but it was some two hours later that I managed to contact her. I receive a good lecture from her!! That it was practically impossible to alter anything at this late stage, unless I wanted to push the costs even higher, I agreed to leave well alone and then if in the future there is another print-run, the alterations can be sorted out then!! So that's how I left it.

Had a short walk, taking it very steady, for now I am getting to the stage where I am almost frightened to stand on the repaired leg at all.

My friend Derrick from just round the corner came in and stayed for an hour just as my meal arrived at 18.20 hours. Scampi, chips and peas with a piece of melon for starters. Hot chocolate later at 20.40 hours. It was after my hot chocolate that I heard Mr Mac was doing his rounds. After a while, when I realised that he was not going to visit, the sister, who I believe had been here all day, came in to say that Mr Mac had not been able to see me but has left orders to say that every other metal stitch can come out tomorrow. Sister tells me, 'He has had a busy day.'

March 22nd

Early start at 6.30 a.m. I have had to send the package back to the printers, also confirming date of delivery for April 2nd—should be home by then??? The night sister had found me some really strong adhesive tape for I wanted it to be nice and secure.

Early morning cuppa 7.30 a.m. with 8.15 a.m. breakfast. Am told it's going to be another busy day for there are twenty new patients coming in today. Toilet, all duties completed, nurse tells me that Cyril next door has been moved to a nursing home.

Oh no, I can't believe it!! While I am reading the paper, a bloodstain appears on the dressing, so I had to ring the buzzer, which, I don't mind telling you, would make me say something under my breath if I was a nurse! But as usual: 'Don't worry, Perc, that's what we're here for.' When staff nurse arrived, change of dressing is accomplished and, having had my mid-morning cuppa, a nurse took me for a short walk. There certainly was lots of activity in and out of the rooms, Mrs Moppses all hot and bothered, for as each patient leaves, perhaps only having been in for a short stay, sometimes as little as two hours, clean linen is the operative word.

Back in 151, staff nurse comes in at 11.30 a.m. to take out every other stitch, then a new dressing is applied. On busy days like today, lunch arrives in due course, yet all waitresses on duty worry that patients will be late getting fed and watered. Yet I know for a fact that some patients infer complaint by saying, 'Tea's late today,' or dinner or lunch come to that! Yes, I recall the chap with a plum in his mouth on a visit to me, who looked at his watch saying, 'The afternoon teas are late today!' And that was only by a few minutes!! It makes me want to spit!!!

Lunch has arrived: CC, various cheeses, tomato and half an onion.

Sheila across the corridor tells me she has varicose veins but is not stopping here. 'Yes, I've had my operation. What are you doing here?' she asked. Like I tell all the others who inquire, 'I caught an infection which has delayed progress.' Margaret next door says she is going home on Sunday, all being well (the lady with the double prosthesis).

During the busy afternoon and early evening, I kept out of the way watching racing from Doncaster even picking out the first winner at 10 to 1.

Sheila has now gone, Mrs Moppses have been in, hovered through and linen is all changed with another occupant installed.

Have a visit from Eric the chap who was in on Christmas Day. It's amazing how much progress he has made, for am certain he could run a marathon already. How he tells me he is able to move about, am sure he is not telling porkies because he looks this sort of chap—with hardly any surplus flesh anywhere. He is a happy chap and quickly has you in fits of laughter.

There is a new agency nurse with us this shift and, after applying a new dressing I decided that she passed with flying colours (myself assessing).

The director in charge of nursing affairs has been called in to have a chat and console a patient who has had a bout of coughing which is persistent, dare I say it, like the gastric problems that I suffered some time ago. This was quickly resolved and, knowing how she beams her personality around you, I bet giving this patient the full treatment soon cured her.

Mr Mac came in: dressing off, has a look at the wound now every other stitch has been removed and says, 'We must get this to heal before I send you home. I'll see you next Saturday.' I wished him well, not knowing where he was going but have noted down, 'Don't know where he has gone, but my god how he has worked this last three weeks. He does deserve a break.'

It sounds as if the head of nurses has also visited another patient beside the one opposite, and guessed she would pop in to see me. Sure thing! She came just as I had started to put a stamp to an envelope. This letter was important because I wanted to catch the last collection. My, wouldn't her dad and Scottie, the chap who would receive this letter in the morning (???) have got on well together for he was a retired Air Force officer with several medals courageously earned, working with the war-time resistance in France. 'Would you like me to post it for you, Percy?' See what I mean!!! Pouring with rain outside (no task difficult if the heart undertakes with generosity) and as usual is dressed as if ready for a dinner engagement. 'I would be grateful if you could, many thanks,' I appreciatively spluttered. She is about to leave when the waitress brings in my tray at 18.15 hours. Straightaway she takes the cover off the main course and discovers lamb chops, cabbage, new potatoes, carrots, mint sauce. Says to the waitress, 'I think it does look good, do you think he will eat all that?' and was gone!!! Wishing me well!!

I have been thinking since I had my meal about what Mr Mac says about me going home, if I am all right, when he comes and sees me next Saturday. If so, then three days later, I should be at home awaiting my delivery of books. I think I shall have to cancel the launch date again.

19.30 hours: the agency nurse comes in to change my dressing after I had called her, for it looked as if the area where it was showing through, the circle, was getting larger. I say to her, 'Don't you think you could squeeze it so it fetches more out? I'll take the blame.' This she did reluctantly, but it certainly moved a fair amount, then a neat dressing was placed over and then I was ready for the night's adventures. I have also noted down that I have lost a lot of blood since I have been in Holly House Hospital.

20.45 hours—hot chocolate with just before lights out—my pills.

March 23rd

7.45 a.m. Early morning cuppa. This is Saturday so today I should get extra cosseting and I guessed correctly. Mind you, there is a staff shortage. Only two waitresses to look after over thirty patients. Breakfast at 8.35 a.m. The nurse who is looking after me this morning, usually works only weekdays, so I know I have to be on my best behaviour. Toilet, usual jobs: staff shortage does not make any difference, as important tasks still have to be done, including having my back washed and dried, and a change of stockings. Cleaning ladies are on top form as well, for when they come in to my room, not only are they sorting out everything that needs it—dusting, hoovering, flowers—but they also make a suggestion that's a complete knock-out: that when I am ready for going home, they want to come and give my home a spring clean! I thanked them most kindly, knowing that I would manage somehow.

Morning cuppa arrived at 11.45 a.m. The trolley lady told me that everywhere is short of staff but not to worry, everybody will be fed some time.

The nursing staff are short-handed as well, for I have made inquiries about my Flucloxacillin pills, knowing they will arrive at some stage. On days like today, I know for a fact that the nurses appreciate you asking them maybe a second time about whatever you might have requested; this jogs a memory lapse, for as I have mentioned before errands are taken on one after the other. They are only human and, with all these patients to look after today, you can imagine what our buzzers are doing to some of their grey cells! Eventually, I got my tablets, a fair time later.

It was 13.00 hours before we had our lunch and for those who did not know how a hospital works when short of staff, the buzzer goes off and it's some time before an answering knock responds on the relevant door. The buzzer is switched off, then inquiries made as to the nature of the call-out. A number of these requests I just cannot print, for it beggars belief what some of them are. I had my usual CC, tomato and a half an onion.

A lady called Kim has come in to find out who the chap is in 151, who has been here for some time. She tells me she has had a Kimberly hip fitted and used to live in Upshire, but now lives in Dorset with her husband and three children, and for most of her life, she has ridden motor cycles. After I told her I had been a motorcyclist myself for well over forty years and had had several accidents, she asked, 'You have been in here some time now, Percy, haven't you?' 'Yes,' I replied, 'I am now called a One-per-center for it stands to reason with all those accidents and the problems that I have had with this infection that we hope is clearing up that the one per cent would finally catch up with me!'

By 14.45 hours, the hospital staff are now back to normal quotas, for as this news came through, the waitress asked me what I wanted with my tea break 'Slice of fruit cake,' I replied, and it arrived at the normal time (I am told) of 15.00 hours.

The senior sister arrives to tell me that she is going to take the last of the stitches out later. I said to her when she gave me this information, 'Good. I am sure it's the metal stitch which is cutting into my leg as I move about so starting it off again.' She looked at me in utter disbelief, saying nothing.

I received a phone call from Patrick, the book agent, telling me that he had received my letter and the date—deliveries were all confirmed. I told him that owing to circumstances here in Holly House Hospital, there might have to be a rearrangement again, but will let him know how things work out. He wished me well, health foremost!! I don't think in all my lifetime that I have not been able to keep appointments as has been the case recently. All those years being my own boss with only two days out!!

Another weekend nurse who has been called in to assist at the pressure points around the wards has arrived to change the dressing and also take the rest of the stitches out. While she was with me, it continued to weep with blood from just the one place. I told her I thought that it was the metal stitch that was pricking me as I moved or walked about. 'I doubt it, Percy,' she said, 'for those stitches are not fixed in a way that would injure patients; they are a vast improvement on the old stitches that I was brought up to deal with. I am on tomorrow, I might suggest an idea to Sister that might work for you in this instance.'

17.00 hours: I am allowed to have a walk along the corridor and back, just with the frame. Sat on the bed and blood started again, so I had to have the dressing changed and made wholesome again. This time, she put a much smaller one around the area causing the most concern.

18.00 hours—steak for dinner and this done—as I have noted down—done beautifully, calabrese, new potatoes with a starter—half a melon.

This was getting annoying for as soon as I had finished my meal so the bleeding started. I dare say, realistically, the size of the area which has to heal makes this a formidable enterprise. If there are five different layers of tissue to heal up following all the major surgeries inflicted on my knee, I suppose the lower ones have to heal properly before the outer and final one says, 'Thank God, this is the last.' I will have to have a word with Chris, my friend the vet, to have this explained a bit more fully, because it does not want to stop bleeding! I had to have another change of dressing soon after the hot chocolate turned up. These two waitresses are what I would call redoubtable tough cookies; they love pulling my leg. I am glad to say that each time they play me up I give as good as I get. I know they love to get me going and I like to wind them up too! And don't expect to find special flaws in their armoury!!! That's true of all the Holly House Hospital personnel! I might also add that you shouldn't think you will get any favours—only if it's seen you are recovering from an operation, when you're entitled to be feeble. Whether or not you like the joviality system, you have to join in with them—or appear to. Then of course you will make great strides in discharging yourself, for much as you love them, they want to see the back of you, make no mistake! Then another success story is chalked up!

They were telling me that the hospital is so busy, that patients are being served pots of teas in the foyer, whilst waiting for a bed; an hour later, all this is under control!!!! No doubt the bridge was working flat out to resolve this situation.

Before my pills arrive, I notice that the big male nurse is on night duty again. But I should imagine he would cope quite well with any problems, as I can already vouch for.

March 24th

Have had a pretty good night—I know I have moved about quite a bit for the sheets are almost on the floor. Unfortunately at 6.50 a.m. I looked at dressing to find blood, so the two night nurses on duty quickly changed the dressing as well as sheets. Felt uncomfortable when the Sunday cuppa arrived. 'Yes,' the waitress says, 'we are coping with all the new arrivals.' There has been some bad news in the sporting world, for one of England's young cricketers has been killed in a car crash, Ben Hollyoake, out in Australia. In New Zealand, England are playing the Second Test, so all test venues around the world are having a minute's silence with the flags at half mast.

10.00 a.m. I am reading my paper when the nurse from yesterday comes in to tell me that she is looking after me and the sister agreed that she could try out her idea to help to stem the flow of blood. I said, 'Go ahead, I'm all yours.'

It's a small round dressing, fits over the cut where the leak is coming from, then sticks all round forming a bag which carries the surplus blood. It's what they call a small colostomy bag. This did not work at first because there was quite a channel which had formed because of all the operations. However, after a couple of adjustments being made and the whole lot taped down, it seemed to work a treat for it was now sealed very effectively. 'We'll see how it goes, then look at it later.'

10.50 a.m. I went for a walk; this was perfect timing, for Kim, the motorcyclist, was just leaving with her family. We all shook hands as if we were long-lost cousins, with a hug or two for good measure.

11.55 a.m.: Derrick, from round the corner comes in, for he knows that, on a Sunday, the lunch is usually a bit special. I always ask him if he will join me, but this he always turns down. It must have made his mouth water, for it was roast beef, Yorkshire, roast potatoes, peas and cabbage. He tells me that a good friend of ours, Doug Insole, the Old Essex and England cricketer has gone to South Africa.

By 14.00 hours when the brains trust nurse came round to have a look, she was over the moon, for the bag had collected a fair drop of blood. You could see she was highly delighted. So I said to her, 'I am going to recommend you for higher office.' 'I've been there, and done that! I'm glad it's worked though. We shall have to keep our fingers crossed. No, I have had my share of that, Perc.'

Next door, 153 has a new patient. She wants to meet me, for one of her friends is or was my neighbour at High Beech, Noreen. Have to have a look in tomorrow.

Another nurse who likes to find flowers for me is having a problem but I tell her, as I have done before—take your time, spend as much time with a patient as you need to; then, when you think there is an improvement starting, you know you have done a great job. That's what your job is all about. The official flower lady is on parade and comes in to say her daughter has fallen over playing netball and sends her love (that's MMM, the young waitress). Of course sent mine by return via Mum. Have noted down, I do envy her granddads. I bet she twists them round each finger. I had another walk to the bridge and back; the bag is holding up nicely and is admired by several nurses as well as staff nurses. I think and say, 'It's magic!'

My evening meal: I am glad that I only ordered a light offering for the CC, cheeses, tomato and onion suited me just right—again though, there were six different types of cream cracker. The cricket match in New Zealand has been drawn.

Hot chocolate came via one of the nurses standing in for a waitress. This is another thing—if it warrants and the trolley needs an extra hand to remove its cargo, the word help is not even mentioned, they just get on with it!

March 25th

6.10 a.m. The staff nurse is round doing observations; she has a good look at the bag which has held up through the night and, as I have noted down, I hope it is leaving off at last. Early cuppa at 7.30 a.m. with breakfast at 8.10 a.m. Had my stockings changed as soon as I had paid my visit to the corner room. This morning I knew the nurse on duty would do my washing—well it's only rinsing out a pair of shorts together with the dirty stockings; legs washed, dried, creamed. Ready for newspaper time, what a life!! No physio!! Still walking with the frame which I can manage reasonably well. Along past the bridge, I am passing the nursing head office and the director says, 'Come in,' after I had knocked on the door of 141 and told her who I was. We had a very pleasant chat, concluding with me mentioning her highly decorative stockings with a diamond pattern on, if I remember correctly. I think she is a great sport.

At lunch I had CC, various cheeses, tomato and half an onion. The early afternoon visitors included the doctor who took some blood, then Lawrence and his wife Debbie who came to see how I was getting on and wondering when I was going to be discharged. I told them as soon as the blood stops and it's beginning to heal. Went for a walk at 16.45 hours, then when I came back a male nurse was now on duty until quite late. I believe it was the first time that he had seen a colostomy bag used for this purpose; in any case, he removed it and replaced it with another one which proved very successful. Observations are usually carried out if possible before evening meals; this time they were completed just before the trolley started its chatter along the corridor: chicken, new potatoes and a salad containing many varieties of mixed goodies. No dessert. Had finished the day with the completion of three letters and making three phone calls. One call I made during the day was to the printers who wanted to know what I thought of the jacket for *Breakout at Sixty-five*. I told him, 'This is something a bit special and yes, it's excellent.'

March 26th

6.00 a.m. Trolley on the move so I know who is in charge, and so there is no sense in doing anything. There was an outstanding letter I wanted to get off so I got stuck into this and finished it before the early morning cuppa arrived at 7.45 a.m. It's a nice bright morning. Breakfast arrived at 8.15 a.m. Then by 9.00 a.m. I had completed all necessary ablutions which included a rinse-out of my pyjama top. Have just started to read the newspaper and, seeing a photo, I thought I recognised that and sure thing it was someone I knew, in the distant past. Unfortunately though, this person had passed away many years ago, for this was her daughter who I was looking at. Talk about the living dead! This person had been kidnapped in Africa, but, fortunately, no harm had befallen her or anyone belonging to this well-known family from Upshire.

10.00 a.m. Pot of tea arrives, then a walk to have a natter to new arrivals. Yes, I have even made some welcome, especially if they seem anxious.

I had several visitors during this period up to the lunch break and then after the lunch interval, there were even more. The morning visitors included Andrew Chilton, another old High Beech family, who had chauffeured Sue over. They stayed for three-quarters of an hour, both wanting to know when I was coming home. I told them exactly as I told others, Mr Mac will not send me home until he is happy with the healing. My observations were done just before the lunch trolley trundled its sweet note along the corridor and my, weren't its contents a bit special—including shrimps, lettuce, tomato, onion—it did look nice.

Pat, Tony, John with a bottle of red wine—I just had a wee dram. It was while we were making merry that John wanted to use the toilet. Of course he got in all right but forgot when he came out that it was a sliding door. There was an almighty crashing noise for it's true, there is nothing on the door to say it slides, but all those standing leapt to his assistance. He had gone the colour of a good crimson globe (beetroot) through his exertions to remove the door completely. You can gather my sides ached with laughter, the same as everyone else. They left at 16.00 hours; everyone who had come in to sample from the paper cups had thoroughly enjoyed a tipple.

My friend Derrick came in. Whilst he was sitting down, the staff nurse came in and drained the blood from the bag, measuring the amount and logging it in my blue book. Had a couple of phone calls as well while he was here. I guessed he was waiting to see what I had got for dinner; then on arrival and removing the lids, 'What's that?'—talk about make your mouth water. Steak and kidney pie, cabbage, asparagus, new potatoes.

19.00 hours went for a walk, then as I was passing the bridge, the phone rang; nurse says, 'It's for you, Percy. Would you like to take it here?' My—I did feel important, taking a message from the main heart of Holly House Hospital.

Through the grapevine, a famous Spurs and international footballer was here and I was going to pass his room—132. Did I dare? No, I chickened out. I still got his autograph though, through one of the staff nurses who was also a Spurs fan, the same nurse who is on duty today. I asked her about the colostomy bag: 'Need I keep it on as there appears to be very little collecting?' The reply: 'We had better keep it on for another couple of days.' Confirmed later with the night senior sister, late in the evening when pills came round.

March 27th

6.00 a.m. Had a pretty good night. Trolley has started up, so I fetched out my pen and paper, and completed a letter to Mr and Mrs Allen in the Forest of Dean, before the early morning cuppa arrived at 7.20 a.m. I asked the head waitress why they are all out of the starting blocks early this morning. 'Yes, we are, Perc,' was her reply. She is a super person—and arranged my birthday bash I'm sure!! Breakfast at 7.40 a.m. Jobs all finished by 8.30 a.m.

Visit from the director of nursing asking me if I would like to move to a room next to her at no 141. 'Yes that's all right with me, that's the one right at the front of the hospital,' I said. 'We like to think it is the best room here,' she answered. I had asked sister if I could have a move some time ago if things didn't improve but my leg is now improving slowly. I told her of my superstitious nature whilst working in the building trade—things like walking under a ladder, number thirteen, etcetera, etcetera.

Between then and 10.45 a.m. I completed a letter to my publisher, also had my colostomy bag removed and dressing applied. Went for a walk along the corridor to talk to a chap who lived at Chingford who knew some customers I had done business with when I was in the building line. We had a rare old chat, lots of past memories. There is also another chap named Geoff, who is going for an operation, so when I told him how long I had been a patient he asked, 'You must be fed up?' 'No,' I truthfully said, 'the time has gone quite quickly for with all those girls buzzing around, you have got to get better.'

11.15 a.m. Back in 151: oh no, oh yes, the bleeding had started again. 'That's because I have been walking along the corridor and chatting I suppose,' I said to the staff nurse who came to change the dressing. Still taking my Flucloxacillin tablet just before my midday meal. CC, various cheeses, tomato and half an onion. It's been confirmed that I have been allotted the Penthouse suite. So at 13.00 hours I start to sort my rubbish out from the locker. Shortly after I had found most of the letters and papers that I wanted to take with me and discarded all that I wanted to bin, Pultzer, the nurse came in to get all my flowers taken to number 141. My, she is a good sport; there doesn't seem anything that's not a problem for her. She says, 'Come on, let's get lively.' I dare say I did seem a bit mesmerised for I had been here in this room, number 151, for sixty plus two days and that's a long time in one room, you must agree? By the time I had walked down to the room with a view for this is what I called it straightaway, I had found that not only were my flowers and pot plants all round the room but new ones as well. 'You're losing your memory, Percy, that's all been brought from your old room!' That was the answer when I inquired as to where they had all come from.

I have noted down—the change has knackered me. Also it has started the blood coming through the dressing, so this has to be changed. I had already looked out of the large mullioned window which overlooked the front entrance, which in turn was also the car park for visitors, outpatients or Holly House Hospital personnel. Fortunately though, I could hardly hear anything for this was a well built property dating back to the nineteenth century. I ought to describe the room—fifteen by fifteen feet with the windowsill a good foot wide. The mullion window was seven foot wide by six foot high. I would guess with the whole of the windowsill maybe, seven foot six inches long and a good foot wide and, like I say, it was packed with flowers. The ceiling height must have been nearly nine feet. Certainly this first glimpse of the room with a view had knocked me for six. 'Come on, Perc, wake up!' The staff nurse had already started and completed draining the nasty coloured liquid which seemed the colour of vinegar.

18.30 hours the trolley with the dinners arrives—scampi, peas and chips, most everybody has been notified that Perc has changed his room number for 141, so it's a continual 'Come in!', 'Whew!' With all the flowers and floral design wallpaper, the room did look nice, and all the nice comments pleased Pultzer even more. The only thing that appears to be giving me quite a bit of annoyance is the bed, for it is making me moan quite a bit! As you can gather I spend a lot of the day on the bed and when I move about this one rocks as if it is going to collapse. I know there is no fear of that but to me it remains unsteady. It's worse when I am being made to laugh which each and everyone does to me whatever their employment here is. After peace and some sort of quietness had returned to number 141, I found that by wedging a chair under the bottom of the bed, it became much more stable. This arrangement was reinforced by the use of the table which has also bonded with the chair, so making sure that any rocking in the bed was reduced to a minimum. I was going to be safe, until the head porter gets to grips with the problems

22.30 hours, the Holly House Hospital flower authority turns up with her daughter (the one who has had an accident playing netball). Straightaway, I have a hug and a kiss, and I have noted down: 'I don't know what Mum thinks, what have they brought in for me??? You guessed it!!—more flowers!! She tells me she is recovering well from her accident and will see us this weekend. Have marked up the diary as well with 'What a day!!!'

March 28th

6.00 a.m. Off to a good start, for the colostomy bag has burst, so I rang for nurse who is only about ten yards along this part of the T-shaped wing of the Holly House Hospital. Sister came in and sorts me out and does a change of sheets; she weighs up the amount of blood left in the bag which is 60 grammes and all is noted down in the blue book. She did remark about the chair and table wedged under the bed, which, as you can guess, did not meet with her approval: 'The sooner I get this changed the better.' I did help her to change the sheets and this did meet with her approval. She suggested that I could soon get a job here if I wanted one.

6.50. am. I started a letter to Sue and completed it by the time that early morning cuppa had arrived.

Breakfast 8.00 a.m. About the bed—have made inquiries of the head porter who is going to sort things out for me a bit later for it's Thursday and operations have already started. So I will have to be patient. Whilst doing my chores in the new toilet, my!—it's twice the size of the one at home, and half as big again as the one I have just vacated.

Out for a walk at 10.15 a.m. Now I am on the same wing of Cedar Ward as Maurice and Geoff. I called in to see them both after my morning cuppa. Both seem a bit down this morning. Geoff, I am sure, has had a rough time, having been brought in as an emergency a few days ago. But like most hospitals, tests have had to be undertaken to confirm what it is that's wrong with him. Now he has had his operation he's had various tests that he is allergic to. He is like me, uncomfortable if the mattress does not fit the posterior. He told me this after I had told him about the problem I had had with my bed and how I had wedged it up.

12.00 hours. Lunch arrives, and also one of the maintenance men who jokingly tells me that this bed is a rocking bed!! Enjoyed my CC, various cheeses with tomato and half an onion, pot of tea.

I went for a walk to number 151 and had a look at the bed I had made vacant. With my good leg, I pumped this up to what I thought was about the right height, thinking that this would suit me, with the same mattress that I had found so comfortable for all those days (mind you, I did get the staff to turn it about several times during this time). While I was on the move I took the lift down to the ground floor and asked permission to look outside as I had not had a good mouthful of air for sixty-one days plus two as I have marked up in my diary. 'Yes, of course you can.' As soon as I was on the ground floor a couple of the waitresses came along and one said, 'Trying to escape, Perc? We are not going to let you go that easily.' I said, 'All I want is some of God's good air.'

Back in the room 141, it's all under control, the bed has been changed over and not only has the mattress been brought with it, but also the donkey pole; as I have mentioned before—what a godsend they are, for levering and manoeuvring in or on the bed. Of course, the removal men had a reward, either chocolate, Polos or similar sweets and I was told it was all completed in ten minutes.

Derrick from round the corner has found me, after he had gone to 151 and found that the room had now got another occupant in. He was told by one of the staff that I had been moved to the penthouse suite. 'What do you think of it?' I inquired.

'I must say you have got some flowers, Perc,' he said, continuing, 'I bet this costs some money.' I said, 'I don't mind where they put me as long as when they do decide on my next move, the next room will be mine at home.'

Towards the end of the afternoon, a staff nurse comes in to say that I am to keep the dressing on below the knee for just a day or two more for it is still weeping a little and maybe the colostomy bag might be changed for an ordinary dressing tomorrow.

The Pultzer Power nurse is on duty on the floor above and of course pops in to see how everything has gone since her help yesterday afternoon. I assured her that lots of people had come in and admired all the decorations.

Dinner at 18.20 hours—shepherds pie, cabbage, new potatoes with a starter of a piece of melon. I had just completed my meal when Mr Philps who is a surgeon at Whipps Cross and also has patients here came in to see me for I am also on his list with other problems. He said, 'I heard you had moved to the penthouse suite. My, it does look nice.' Whilst he was with me talking I told him that I was visiting one of his patients along the corridor named Maurice. 'Splendid, good man, he needs cheering up.' During the rest of the evening I have several staff come to visit me and all enthuse over the room with a view. All the get-well cards are likewise now in their right places and all have been acknowledged. It was later that the night staff came in and emptied the colostomy bag. This measured 60 grammes.

March 29th

Early start at 6.30 a.m. I could hear the trolley about, so I got out of bed and drew the curtains and tied them back with the special ribbons attached. The senior night staff (Annie Get Your Gun) came in and removed the colostomy bag, this time for good, replacing it with a dressing. There was a small amount of blood which looked a healthier colour. She also tells me as it is Easter weekend, she and a few more nurses are taking some handicapped children to Lourdes. Would I like her to say a prayer for me? 'Yes of course I would.' This agreed, the senior sister came in with a pair of scissors. A lock of my hair was cut off and taken away. Pultzer Power nurse comes in to say she is looking after me all day. There have been several admissions during the night—I thought this might be the case for as I have mentioned before I am now near where all the action takes place.

Breakfast at 8.15 a.m. Then usual duties including sorting

out some bloodstained shorts that have been contaminated, presumably by the colostomy bag, It has not leaked anything since I have had the new dressing on. Of course, the sheets are changed again—so by 10.15 a.m. I went to walk the corridors. First a visit to Maurice who seems a lot better this morning. Well he had a good laugh at a few of the tales I was telling him. Unable to travel anywhere else as the carpet cleaners are on the main Cedar Ward. I took the lift up to the second floor and saw several nursing staff and admin personnel who all inquired after my health, wondering when I was going home. I told them, 'I am sure it won't be long now.' The terrible twins were also on duty—they could see that I was making good progress. I had not seen Ted for some time; he tells me he is into his twelfth day—he's the chap who had a double knee operation.

Lunch break—12.00 hours. Piece of fried cod, chips and peas. The afternoon I did not move far as I watched football on Sky between 14.00 and 16.00 hours. Whilst I was out having a walk I had a chat with the carpet cleaners who tell me that they have to clean the carpets along and outside 141. I asked them, 'What time do you expect to finish?' for it was now nearly 17.00 hours and this wing had not even been started. I inquired about assistance. 'Help, no there are only the two of us and we should get it completed by 22.00 hours.

While I was moving around I called in to Geoff's who tells me that his mattress has been changed and is now much more comfortable. Knowing he was a keen sportsman, I asked him what he thought of the match this afternoon. We both agreed that Bobby Robson, since he has been at Newcastle, has certainly improved the team. Seems a lot better. I have told him when he is up and about he will have to come and see my room, for compared with this one, mine is three times as big and just oozes quality.

Dinner arrives at 18.30 hours. As I had enjoyed my meal earlier, I had ordered CC, various cheeses, tomato and half an onion.

About 19.30 hours: it's gone pretty quiet outside. The carpet cleaners have done a runner and gone home, finished? No, coming back another time.

I have another new neighbour who is next door at 138 (yes, that is correct, 138); her name's Joan and I mentioned before she is a friend of my old neighbours at High Beech, Noreen and Ian. So I ring her up to find out if it's convenient for me to pop in to see her. Sorry she is watching one of her favourite programmes—*Morse*. I said, 'I'll call another time.'

Late hot chocolate with, just before lights out, pills including change of dressing, clean up.

March 30th

I have noted down straightaway before the day's activities get under way—must mention the sunset last night. It's a long time since I saw one like that. Magic!!

I have been awake since well before 6.00 a.m. The trolley starts up, in fact a couple of times, can't really say what the interruption is but it could have been a nearby buzzer going off.

After my observations have been done, I start a letter and complete it by the time early morning cuppa arrives. I did not enjoy my cuppa for just prior to this, the sister came in and took a swab from the place where the blood is coming from. After, of course, drying the whole area and making it look presentable she said it's important to take one for Mr Mac wants to see this later.

I was surprised to see how far she penetrated the wound. As I remarked, it must have been a good inch. Her reply: 'Yes,

I would think so, looks as if you will be leaving about the same time as me, in about three weeks time.' I said, and thought at the time, 'Oh my god! Perhaps my Annie Get Your Gun has not arrived at Lourdes yet!' So I keep my fingers crossed that the prayer has not gone through yet but will be answered when it does. 7.30 early morning cuppa. Knock on the door—7.45 a.m. Mr Philp asks, 'Did you see that catch of Graham Thorpe's?' (Like me—interested in cricket.) He is here to visit patients.

Breakfast at 8.15 a.m. Wash, shave, all jobs completed by 9.00 a.m.

I am still not able to do any exercises as it has been pointless to do any for it will only start the wound off again and at this late stage I don't want any aggravation starting. Morning cuppa at 10.15 a.m. and at 10.40 a.m. went for a walk, just to see how much of an improvement the carpet men had made yesterday—after seeing where they had completed. It's amazing how different it looked, which must have given a lot of satisfaction all round. Called in to Maurice, who had the two ladies with him whom I had seen before. So politely I said, 'I'll call another time.'

At 12.25 hours, the MMM waitress arrives with CC, various cheeses, tomato and half an onion.

Mr Mac calls in with the senior sister, the dressing is removed. I shake his hand, asking him if he enjoyed his trip. 'Yes,' he said, adding, 'It's healing nicely.' I asked him how things stood re going home: 'For as you are aware, I have the most important date in my life coming up in just over three weeks time at the Epping Bookshop and I don't want to cancel any more.' Mr Mac says, 'As soon as I see the results of the swab and if it's okay, you will be able to go home on Wednesday.' While he was with us I did make him laugh, for I told him about my cousin Dickie, who on my instructions had removed my dahlia tubers from their winter storage in the electric meter cupboard under the neighbour's staircase. Vital! I was a bit concerned that if I left them there, they, the neighbours up top, might be cutting the blooms before me and that would not do.

The two ladies who had visited Maurice came in to see 'the room with a view', staying only a couple of minutes. As they were leaving, one said, 'Cheerio, Percy Blakeney.' As I knew they were both acquainted with the Redcliffes of Chingford, I told them that I had built an arched opening at his Gresham works in Chingford and he had named it 'Percy's Portal'. This made them both laugh as they left Room 141.

Did not do much the rest of the afternoon, football game between Leeds (3) and Manchester United (4). Watched the racing, then a walk up to second floor, each time I came back to 141, the phone rang asking me where had I been—one person thought that I might have gone home.

By 17.30 hours, my observations have been done, everything is up. My temperature has a reading of under 37!! That's okay.

Dinner arrives 18.30 hours. Fried fish, peas and chips. An apple.

Derrick is late coming in today. He did not arrive until nearly 17.00 hours, so he could not see what it was that I had under the stainless steel covers. However when I told him, he said, 'I bet it was nice,' looking at the plate, which did not need any washing up! As I was feeling pretty good I walked down with him to the foyer and saw him off the premises. I was surprised how well he seemed tonight for he handled his walking stick quite ably just as I was coping reasonably well with mine. I noticed one thing as we opened the door. My, it was cold outside tonight! The last bit of news for the day that I have recorded is that the Queen Mum has died at 15.15 hours.

March 31st, Easter Sunday

One of the first things that went through my mind when I got up at 8.00 a.m. was that I did not expect to be here in Holly House Hospital on Easter Sunday.

The clocks had gone forward one hour, so the night sister had come in with a screwdriver to alter the clock. This though was the wrong size—much too small for whatever she had to do. I asked her, 'Are you a do-it-yourselfer?' 'Why of course!' was her reply. Then, realising that it was best for her to seek help, she said, 'I'll be back in a few minutes.' It did not take much longer than that, telling me all she had to do was take the rim off and move the hands. This quickly done, the clock now read 8.15 a.m. That only took ten seconds for I said I would time her as to the length of time it took. Of course, she was rewarded with some chocolates. I had already had my early morning cuppa, then breakfast at 8.20 a.m.

9.30 a.m. enter the toilet, had nearly completed all my tasks, when I noticed blood on the floor!! Oh no!! Wound had opened up again and the night sister had had a look at it only about an hour and a half ago and it was dry for we both remarked how well it looked (of course under the dressing). It's so disappointing. I really did think that I had seen the last of the blood. Not so!! And you would never believe who was on duty to come and sort it out for me. Yes, you have guessed it, the same staff nurse who was on duty with the other bloody episodes in room 151.

'What have we been up to now then, Perc?' she said as she entered 141.

I said, 'It's some weird blood this time. Take a look at it, it's the colour of Sarsons vinegar. It looked strange the other day, but how about that?' Of course, it's all in a morning's work to her for it was tidied up with a new dressing, sheets changed in no time and I'm soon looking respectable again. Have been reading the Sunday newspaper, and of course it's full of the Queen Mum. I decided to do some walking so first up to the second floor, then along the corridor of Cedar ward. While I am out, I pop in to see Maurice and Geoff, who tells me that he is so much more comfortable with the mattress that had been changed due to the newly formed patients' association which managed to get things moving right from the very top, myself Chairman!!! We certainly had a good laugh.

The weekend Mrs Moppses are in good form this morning for the MMM is on duty!!! When she is not causing blood pressure with her waitress duties around the wards, she fills in with Mrs Moppses' duties and yet still has time to pop in to see how I am getting on. I tell them my days are numbered for sure. 'When are you going home, Perc?' 'I'll let you know!' Shortly after this, dressing changed again with same colour blood.

12.00 hours—roast turkey, roast potatoes, Yorkshire, cabbage, peas, an apple.

Saw, during the afternoon, some of the Queen Mum's life. It seems to me she helped the old King George VI's reign to prosper more than I had ever imagined. Oh well, you generally find out some time about royalty and its ups and downs through the years.

16.30 hours. Another leak, same sort of blood with another new dressing, this time nurse applied dressing just with the gauze taped down. Looking at the old one, lot of blood and muck. Nice and tidy once more, went for another toddle, but still I have not been told I can do the staircase. I suppose this is sensible thinking for though I know I would take it carefully, I am not the one making decisions. I have opened my package which arrived this morning—one large Easter egg with the compliments of Holly House Hospital. There are not many patients on the second floor so I take the lift down to the ground, this time having a chat with one of the reception girls who knows the Howes' family from Loughton. Decide to phone my old pal in Somerset and ask him how he is keeping and if he's happy with the cricket in New Zealand.

18.10: trolley is moving with meals on wheels service, delivers to me a magnificent piece of salmon, with this a huge salad, new potatoes and a piece of melon for starters.

I know I might get some visitors soon or tomorrow, so rang the ones who I thought might be visiting to tell them that I am now in room 141. I also rang my own Mrs Mopps at home to ask her if she would be so kind as to take my curtains down and give them a good wash. The reply, 'Yes that's all right, Perc'.

The night sister came in later; she noticed that I was doing some exercises but nothing too strenuous for I did want to impress Mr Mac that it was my intention to try to make the Wednesday D-Day discharge.

April 1st, Easter Monday

I had turned the cricket on at 5.15 a.m. New Zealand were struggling and by 5.45 a.m. they were all out for 202 runs and England at 7.10 a.m. was not faring too well for they were 12 runs for 3 wickets.

The night staff have had to change the sheets, also the dressing, same colour blood. Sister pops in to say don't do any bending at all—it must heal. Of course it's April Fool's Day, so I thought I would try some of the nurses and staff to see if they were awake. One or two of the waitresses were caught out when sent to see some ambulances arrive outside on the drive, only to look through the window to find nothing there. 7.30 a.m. April fooled!! Early morning cuppas and breakfast a bit later at 8.10 a.m. Then the Mrs Moppses' turn. I pretended that I was talking to someone in my old room 151, as, walking past it, I could see there was no one there. A couple working in a nearby room said to each other, 'Who's he talking to, there's no one in 151.' Sure thing they came up to find the room indeed was empty. April fooled. But it was not long before they had their own back, asking me if they knew Lawrence had come in suddenly and wanted to see me. Of course, I fell for it hook, line and sinker. April fooled.

Scissors is looking after me this morning so I knew that I would have not only my back attended to but also get a change of stockings, both legs sorted out and both creamed; both legs and feet have had to have a good soaking first before the gentle massage. She has come up with a good idea and I'm pretty sure I have not mentioned this before. Where I had my leg brace on just behind my ankle, where the bottom part of brace is, as I moved around it had formed a slight wound which had almost healed, leaving a scab which might bleed and that would not do; so, before the stockings were put on, a dressing was placed over it, which hopefully would not hinder the healing process. Then the stockings were very carefully put back on. Magic!

The physiotherapist pops in to see me: 'Orders are to let it heal before any exercise is applied.' I told her, 'I am getting concerned that my leg is never going to be straight again; when can I start trying to bend it?' 'No worry, once you start bending it, it won't take long to get your leg as good as the other one. You have to give it time.'

Morning cuppa at 10.45 a.m.

When I saw most of the Mrs Moppses again, each party was wary of the other's remarks, for it wouldn't do to be caught too often. Several of the smart staff I tried to add to my victims, but to no avail. I was told by one that I had got some visitors waiting in 141 but as this was confirmed by a couple of other nurses, I realised that this was genuine. Sure thing—my cousin Keith and his wife. They stayed for an hour or so, leaving just before my lunch arrived at 12.15 hours: CC, various cheeses, tomato and half an onion.

As you realise I am a very fidgety person and as I had completed all my correspondence, there was no need to keep lying on top of my bed so I walk to the top floor via the lift, walked the top corridors, then Cedar Ward, finally popped in to see Geoff who is an Arsenal supporter. Spurs were on the television this afternoon, KO at 14.00 hours. I watched the match from my room and, while it was on, the male nurse came in to change the dressing. It all looks pretty good with just this one area where the weeping is coming from. Colour is, I would say, back to normal. Tottenham (2) Leeds (1) was the football result.

My friend Derrick, came in and I did not think he looked at all well for he was very unsteady when he sat down, nearly toppling over. I asked him if he had watched the football. 'No, I can't be bothered,' he said. I soon cheered him up when I told him of some of the April 1st capers I and others had been involved with. One thing we both agreed was that it had been a nice Easter Monday. He left at 5.45. I was surprised that he went before my dinner had arrived for, as I have mentioned, he likes to see what is hidden under the covers. This time it was roast pork, peas, cabbage, roast potatoes and new ones as well. I did have a starter—half a melon.

I have a visit from Doreen, Maurice's wife, who tells me that he is going home tomorrow. Then, no sooner than the door had closed my friend the vet, Chris comes in. My—I don't mind telling, again I was given a lecture on how my knee should be progressing, the reasons why progress is slow and why it is not a normal straightforward major operation as prostheses go. I only wish sometimes I could tape the knowledge that comes from her grey cells. She has had a busy day driving her land rover all over the fields beside Gravel Hill, pulling some harrows, this to aerate the coming new season's grass. The senior sister comes in to see how I was. I told her I am sure changing the room has made all the difference. 'I doubt it, Percy, but you have only been in a few days and probably going home Wednesday so that's good.' 'Do you think it's all right for the barber to cut my hair before I go home?' 'Yes, of course, if she is not too busy. Mind you, when I saw her this morning, she seemed as if she was brewing for a cold.'

Hot chocolate and tablets, with lights out at 23.00 hours.

April 2nd

I am awake at 5.00 a.m. so I turned on the cricket from New Zealand. It seems as if England are struggling. Early morning cuppa at 7.30 a.m. Breakfast at 8.15 a.m. Have completed all my jobs and though I have had a visit from the night staff, the dressing is dry and does not appear to be leaking. At 9.30 the nurses come in to sort this all out together with a change of linen. I thought myself it seemed a lot better all the way down my leg, not healthy like the other leg, but there was a get-up and go about it surely, I kept kidding myself. Have had several visitors this morning including Sue, her son Julian and Tania who are pleased to hear that I might be going home tomorrow. Then a familiar face of some fifteen years ago walked past. Instantly I called out, 'Is that you, Pat?' Yes, indeed, it was one of our footballers' wives of some eighteen years ago. She told me after a big hug that Stewart, her husband, was in here with a slipped disc, just along the corridor in Room 149. I then met one of the two daughters who now was not only a mum herself but Stew and Pat were grandparents. Whew!!

Maurice is off shortly and tells me that he is eighty-two and has so much enjoyed our company.

Geoff at 137 has been watching cricket for he is still not able to move about following his operation but seems a cheerful chap, telling me, 'The result between the two countries could go three ways. A draw, a win for us or a win for them—New Zealand.' Lunch at 12.20: CC, various cheeses, tomato and half an onion.

Scissors comes in this afternoon and tells me that she has brought the scissors with her but is working on the top floor and it's pretty busy but will do my hair if it's possible—she will see how it works out.

What I did do was shortly after lunch I went up and asked the sister in charge if Scissors could weigh me. 'Yes certainly, Perc.' I weighed in at one pound less than when I stood on them not so long ago. I could hardly believe this for Scissors seemed taken aback by my doubting of the scales and her interpretation.

Back in Room 141, I completed reading the second of my birthday presents about Jim Laker's life. My—what a player he was! I am pretty sure this is only the second cricket book that I have ever completed following the Brian Johnson story back in late February, both great stories.

Pultzer nurse is with me now during this afternoon and evening rota. I am confident she will graduate in this profession—and undoubtedly will progress under the guidance of so many excellent staff nurses—for to me she seems to have a positive attitude, something that each member of this profession has in buckets. I get the impression there is always a deep conscience, within each and everyone's intellect, whereby tasks are taken on board—errands, fetch a pill, pick a message up, in a minute, a couple or even five—can you give me a hand? I need help. In whatever order they are received, they are still logged, and when that grey matter clicks in ('Remember so-and-so'), then there is a response and the job is carried out. Very few patients understand or realise that whatever the hospital—be it private or NHS—that the nurse has only one pair of hands, and she will eventually attend to your needs.

No, I don't want any medals or bonus points for making this disclosure— it's been going on since beds were introduced into hospitals all those generations ago. I have seen this amazing recall on umpteen occasions, and am sure others will have witnessed this as well.

I dare say what gives me confidence to make this observation is the fact that I am now into my sixty-eighth day of being an eyewitness to all this good will. I have seen with my own two eyes. Yes, I have benefited from little gifts, paid from their own pockets in some instances, with never a thought of reimbursement. Those favours have been acknowledged and appreciated, welcomed and received in the same spirit as the big-hearted benefactor intended. As I get into this mode of thought, it's amazing how so many good Samaritan efforts and gestures over this long period of hospitalisation come flooding back to me—the times staff were running errands, doing good turns, not only for me, but other patients that I was in close contact with. Sometimes in their break times, sometimes while completing official duties, a host of kindnesses—stamps envelopes, fruit, bottles of mineral water, the list, as I recall, is endless; nearly forgot—flowers, pot plants and the like.

During the afternoon, the staff nurse came in and changed my dressing. My—was there some horrid muck discharging! Anyhow, soon tidied up with fresh dressing applied, then walking, exercises, second floor to see the barber. It seems neither of us are able to fit this trim in because she is busy and I am really waiting for Mr Mac to pop in to see me and tell me the good news.

It was after Derrick had come and gone, I had eaten my dinner—scampi, chips and peas that at 18.45 hours Mr Mac came in to say, 'Yes, it's all right for you to go home tomorrow,' asking me if it's sorted out at home. Before I go he wants me to collect pills, further dressings and a letter for the district nurse who will have to keep an eye on the wound, adding, 'We will make an appointment for next Wednesday the 10th. Keep using the walking stick,' again emphasising that I must let it all heal and no bending of the knee—that is important. I told him, 'I am concerned about the bending of the knee, only it is now nearly four weeks since I have done any work with the knee exercises.'

'Not to worry, I have told you, if we can't get it to bend, I will bring you in for a day, send you to sleep and manipulate it on the power machine.'

I then made several phone calls, including one to the lady who was going to wash my curtains.

'Sorry, Perc, Pat is ill, so I am unable to do them.' I then had a walk saying to different people that this was the last evening stroll I was taking as I was most certainly going home tomorrow.

Hot chocolate and pills later. Lights out after completing another and hopefully my last letter from this address, c/o Holly House Hospital.

April 3rd

Have turned the telly on at 5.45 a.m. and Ceefax tells me that England have lost the test match by 78 runs, having been set 312 runs to win—all out 233.

Early morning cuppa at 7.00 a.m. with breakfast at 7.55 a.m., then followed a fair bit of time sorting out all the rubbish again which I had collected in just the seven days I have been here. As there was a television replay of the final day's play between New Zealand versus England, I watched right through to 9.25 a.m. The little dark nurse who is one of those with a very deep conscience has brought me a tablet which for some reason went missing some time ago, assuring me time and time again that it is not her fault, really taking this to heart. Again this is another example of dedication. I said, 'Don't worry, I knew that I would get it before long.' A whisper has reached me that eighteen patients are coming in today so you may depend the room with a view would not be unoccupied for very long. Staff nurse changed dressing, stockings, etc. I said to her, 'I hope they give me plenty of dressings.' Was the aperture getting smaller? So Chris the lady who I had met back in September was now here again for another operation in 148. She helped me pack most of my things including some of the pot plants which found their way into carrier bags.

At 10.30 a.m. I started saying my goodbyes, which included showing to a few of the admin staff the advance information sheet on my book *Breakout at Sixty-five*. My—weren't they surprised!! All wishing me the best of luck with it, I told them that the launch date would be later this month. Saw my old footballer, Stew and his wife Pat, told them about the book, they both wished me well with it. Saw Geoff further along at 137. Like me, he was a bit disappointed with England's cricket results. It then was time to say ta-ta, hugs and kisses to all the staff with handshakes for the porters. Then down below. My—what a send-off! Most of the staff had come to give me a hug and a kiss. I told them that they were all a super bunch and I had never been treated like this before.

'Your taxi's here, Perc,' and I was gone also with my hanky out—like some of the girls in the foyer.

Reaching home at 12.10 when something like ten children all shook my hand—asking me if I had come home to stay.

The following staff are names that I became acquainted with during my long stay at Holly House Hospital;-

Mr McAuliffe's secretaries, Trish and Jo.
Director of Nursing
Sisters: Brenda, Penny, Janet, Diane, Tiggie
Staff Nurses: Gemma, Jane, Linda, Lesley, Leslie-Anne, Lorraine, Sally Snr, Sally Jnr, Kathy,
Tina, Sue, Carol, Cicelle, Sylvia, Helen, Margrina, Fiona, Val, Margaret, Vicky, Rose-Marie.
Nurses: Diane, Joan, Janet, Margo, Ringo, Philly, Stephanie, Elaine, Marline. Jo, June
Male nurses: Moses, June, Feman, Graham, Christian.
Waitresses: Lorraine, Shirley, Yvonne, Rita, Sue, Sandra, Irish, Leah, Lou
Mrs Moppses: Barbara, Pat, Barbara, Maureen, Marg, Wendy, Sarah
Weekend Mrs Moppses: Jade, Clare, Lou
Porters: Bill. Denis, Paul.
Physios: Gill, Anne, Chris, Jenny, Caroline, Donna, Bev, Helen
Pharmacist: Mrs T T
Outpatients Nurses: Sheena, Mary, Carol, Jenette
Administration: Jenna, Jane, Jackie, Marion
Accounts: Chris, Amanda, Mary
Reception: Chris, Sue, Chris, Linda
Maintenance chaps: Gareth, Harry

My nick names for some of the staff who I considered worthy of their titles—were as follows: two RSMs (Regimental Sgt Majors), Sprinter, Scissors, Pultzer (My little nicotine girl), 3MMM, Big B, Gert and Dais, plus the Terrible Twins).

I'm sure there are names I have missed out, but I feel proud that I have remembered so many, for as most of the staff know, I was often capable of making mistakes. If you're not listed, you can be sure I think you are just as important as those mentioned.

When I arrived home, I thought that it would only be a week or so before I could do all those things that I had promised myself I would be indulging in. Not so!!! Contacting the local district nurse, I am informed that she is coming in to see me tomorrow morning to carry on with the good work of rehabilitation. Am cutting my diary down to size now with brief accounts of most days' exploits.

April 4th

The district nurse arrived at 11.30 a.m. and replaced the dressing that I had put on the night before. There had been quite a bit of discharge; she asked me, 'Can you walk? If so you can walk as far as the paper shop. Take it steady as we don't want to make the wound any worse.'

'Yes of course I can,' I replied.

April 5th

Nurse called at 10.00 a.m. Took off all the old dressing and replaced it with a waterproof one. This nurse, I must say, had miles of paperwork which did not help, taking down all my history as I was added to the seemingly endless pages, leaving a prescription for me to collect more dressings. I will mention that as today has been a super day (weather-wise) have enjoyed it immensely. I changed the dressing at 23.00 hours with wound—no change.

April 6th

Nurse called 11.30 a.m. This morning there has been a fair bit of discharge. She also did me a favour by changing my stockings (must get the hang of these). Bedtime, change of dressing—still the same colour.

April 7th

The nurse who changed my dressing for the waterproof ones I was having to put on, put a probe into the aperture, measuring it. I agreed that it was one inch and a quarter deep. Of course, there was much more blood and pus coming out, for I distinctly heard it pop. As everyone tells me, from the sisters, nurses in the hospital and now the district nurse inform me: It's better out than in!!! Change of dressing before bedtime.

April 8th

Two nurses called at 10.45 a.m. The senior one of the two, no doubt, having read through my notes, decided to pack some seaweed into the hole where the discharge is oozing from. This, I am informed again, certainly helps the healing process. I changed the whole lot before I went to bed sealing the whole with the waterproof dressing.

April 9th

When I got out of bed this morning, I found that the seaweed plug was lying on the bedroom floor, so it must have squeezed out somehow. So rang the surgery when they opened and asked if I could come down and have it attended to. I was finding walking much easier with the walking stick so about 11.00 a.m.

I left home taking it steady, arriving just before my appointed time of 12.00 hours. After Dr Wong and the nurse had looked at the hole, on his instructions, she packed more into the aperture, then a gauze dressing with a plain one finally all sealed down with Microtape. Am leaving the whole of the dressings on, trusting that I don't move about too much in the night.

April 10th

Am happy with the situation when I got up, so decided to leave well alone until Mr Mac sees it later on in Outpatients at Holly House Hospital.

I completed my cooking session by late morning and carefully placed the results in tinfoil with three in tins of the right dimensions, these to be delivered when I arrived later. These few Victoria sponges are my way of saying thank you for all the TLC I received and though I say it myself with home-made blackberry jelly filling, they did look the part!! Arriving at Holly House Hospital I was soon spotted by my old friends who quickly gave me a hug and a kiss. I went straight into the kitchen where I collected some more; no doubt, the staff here have been forewarned that I was delivering edible goods. 'You didn't make these, Perc, did you?' each one asked.

Mr Mac has a look at the wound and seaweed tucked in, now exposed for all to see.

'As I don't like seaweed being used to help wounds to heal, we'll remove this straightaway,' and said to the nurse, 'I would like you to take a swab before you put the fresh dressings on.'

April 11th

I went to the surgery by bus at 12.15 hours. Saw the nurse, explaining that Mr Mac did not approve of seaweed for healing purposes. 'That's all right with us. The surgeon has the last word and we only follow instructions.' She then tidied it up with a new dressing in place. I have marked down in today's notes: 'Am sure I am improving but have lots of aches and pains, lower region of back. Important phone calls today.' The phone calls were made. I had realised for some time that April 25th was out of the question for a book launch and it would have to be postponed. The new date May 2nd seemed to suit all the parties involved, the publisher, the printer, the agent who gets the books to various outlets up and down the country and chiefly myself. So it must be for the best, because I wanted to go and sign copies of my book in a much better frame of mind than at present. This period gives me another three weeks.

April 12th

Up at 7.00 a.m. Bottom sheet is a right mess, so tidied up the part where discharge is coming from with the new dressings supplied. I replace the waterproof dressing replaced, spray pads with sterile saline aerosol to make sure that my wound continues in the right direction, then finally seal all this with the Microtape. The latter part of the day, I have dunked them both (lower part of legs) in the bath and changed my DVT stockings. When I changed my dressing later, I have noted down—wound is closing fast (healing that is).

April 13th

7.00 a.m. Wound is still discharging so did the usual, making it all wholesome again, with fresh dressing.

I am now back to driving my vehicle, as I have met with Dr Wong's approval for this. It's made a big difference for the buses, though they are promised every twenty minutes, whenever

I use them, this is certainly not the case. Kept the dressing on for rest of day and did not even change it at bedtime.

April 14th

There is a strong wind blowing today but showers are forecast as well according to the weathermen at 7.00 a.m. Later, find out he was almost correct. The wound has made very little discharge so just made it all look respectable again. I know yesterday was the 13th day of the month but could this have warranted a change for the better, as you must have come to realise I avoid bad luck days like the plague—but is there a wind of change about? Yes I have made a note to this effect. We shall see.

April 15th

7.00 a.m. As the dressing shows no discharge, decide to keep it in place. I have an appointment with the nurse at the surgery this morning at 11.00 a.m. Arriving at the surgery, the nurse told me that the swab they had taken earlier last week was good so she tidied it up and replaced with an ordinary sterile dressing. It certainly looks more healthy so perhaps the corner has been turned. I did some tying in with my trained blackberry this afternoon and found several that were in blossom, have noted down this must be a record—middle of April and blossom from a bramble.

April 16th

Up at 7.00 a.m. I changed the dressing—does not look too good this morning for there has been a discharge from that very same hole. Still I have to see Mr Mac tomorrow afternoon, so see what he says. I have received a message to say that the staff have all enjoyed the Victoria sponges at Holly House Hospital.

April 17th

As there does not appear to be any leakage from the wound I have decided to leave the whole lot in place, then Mr Mac can see for himself what has collected in the hours prior to the new dressing being applied. My appointment was for 15.00 hours. The Outpatients' nurse removed all the old dressing which to my mind did not look too bad, though the liquid discharging certainly looked a funny colour. When he saw it, he told me that swab they took last Wednesday showed that I had another growth, so I would have to go on another course of antibiotics: 'Come and see me next Wednesday and we'll see how it has progressed.' So he gave me a prescription which I later collected from Dr Wong.

April 18th

I am so glad that the book launch date has been rearranged. For this morning when I got up round about 7.00 a.m. it did not feel right under the dressing. Sure thing! Filthy gungy stuff was coming out from the hole, now fractionally larger. After taking the new pills through the day and last one just before bedtime, it might be helping the growth to improve. What it certainly was doing was curing my aches in the groin, back, hip (left side) other knee!!! Could hardly feel any pain at all.

April 19th

Up at 7.00 a.m. I changed the dressing straightaway, looking at wound which had improved very substantially, even, I thought, the colour. Mind you, the weather outside had been pretty dismal, as it must have rained all night, according to the puddles that are around as I went to get my paper.

My appointment with the nurse was for 10.30 a.m. She gave it a good clean-up and put a new dressing on, also finding some more replacements. She also did me a favour changing the old stockings for the clean ones I had brought with me. I'd hoped that she would be kind enough to do the honours. 12.30: Lyn the printer delivers 500 books; *Breakout at Sixty-five* is here at last! I changed the dressing later to find the same colour discharge.

Saturday, April 20th

When I changed the dressing at 7.00 a.m. there was a fair bit of discharge. I have noted down, 'When's it going to stop?' Kept it on all day, changed it last thing at night.

April 21st

Up at 7.15 a.m. There has been more discharge, seems to be the same colour and substance as earlier!!!!! 'HOPE IT'S NOT!!!!!' I have marked down in big capitals. I am now also getting lots of pain again, groin, lower part of back. My cousin, Dickie arrived to take the dahlia tubers up the garden. Not to plant—to harden them off. I hardly helped at all for I ached all over, and was glad when this task was completed. Later I went up and covered them with nets, in case of night frosts. These are a bit special for I have been growing them now (same variety) for over twenty years. So I don't want to lose them.

Later, last thing, changed the dressing.

April 22nd

Up at 7.00 a.m. Sure thing!!! There has been a frost, nothing special but just to warn people not to be too hasty, because Jack Frost can be a nasty temperamental old devil when he wants to be as I have found out during a lifetime of dealing with him.

Rang the nurse at the surgery to find out if she could see me this morning! 11.30 a.m. 'That's fine,' I said.

When I was called in to see her, I told her that it had been discharging all over the weekend. Good clean-up operation with a new dressing, also a prescription for some more sterile dressings. Left this one on until I changed it just before bedtime.

April 23rd

I am doing a few exercises each morning on the bed before I remove the old dressing as I feel if I don't I might never be able to bend it again, but have to be careful how I do those exercises, just short and gentle ones and am sure they are doing no harm at all.

This morning, after I had completed them, I changed the dressing; it's been discharging again. There has been quite a bit of rubbishy coloured muck coming out—in fact, a vinegary shade. All tidied up, fresh dressings applied but still have plenty of aches and pains in back, groin, both legs. I did not interfere with it any more until bedtime, when I replaced everything.

April 24th

Have to see Mr Mac this afternoon so decided to leave the dressing on, as it seems to be dry with no discharge from anywhere.

The aches and pains have got no better. I suspect that it was all sixty-eight days of reduced activity causing this; you don't realise how harmful this is going to be in the long-term. You never give this idleness a second thought when your body parts are crying out for movement of some description (your muscles). Should I have tried a bit harder? No I mustn't say that for all of the physio ladies say that most of the time I wanted to push on with workouts if warranted.

The first words Mr Mac said when he saw me at the appointed time were, 'Many thanks for the book,' which he had received from me, telling me that he had not had time to read it but was looking forward to it. Then his next words were, 'I might have to cut you open again, near where the wound is discharging.' After he had given the whole leg an inspection I exclaimed, 'Oh dear!' Completely taken by surprise, I was lost for words, letting this short sharp sentence be slowly absorbed with its implications. The Outpatients' nurse on duty says she is also surprised that it is taking such a long time to heal, continuing, 'Let's keep our fingers crossed.' I then reminded her that as Mr Mac assures me I am a one-per-center, this is why it is still continuing, I am sure.

Left the dressing on for the rest of the day.

April 25th

At 7.00 a.m. there has been a fair bit of discharge; cleaned, redressed, tidied up and made everywhere wholesome again. As I apply each new dressing, I keep saying to myself, 'Where on earth does all this mucky stuff come from?' When I was tying in the blackberries yesterday, I scratched myself and it was beautiful blood. Changed the dressing last thing at night, it has discharged just a little but am sure the colour is not so nasty looking.

April 26th

Have to see the nurse this morning at 11.00 a.m. Up my usual time—7.00 a.m. Not a very good morning as it's raining and forecast for most of the day.

Saw the nurse at a few minutes past the hour who seemed quite pleased with the wound and after tidying it all up remarked, 'It looks as if an improvement is on the way.' It might have been the colour of the muck that was coming out or maybe the look of the whole width of the scar; in any case, she made me look at it quite differently. If she was happy with the situation, so should I be.

I have still got the aches and pains all around the lower regions including my back and have taken some painkillers for those which unfortunately do not click in just like putting your foot on the throttle pedal, you have to wait and be patient, but in any case it should be worth the wait. During the afternoon, I washed and had a good scrub up along with a change of DVT stockings. These are changed every other day.

April 27th

I have done something today that I am indeed very proud of!!! I have sold some books and done another book signing!!!

Had not done anything with dressing during the whole day for it did not warrant changing, I considered. Even my pains and aches were not quite so noticeable and then of course the moment I thought about them, they seemed to multiply in no time. However at 23.00 hours I changed the dressing, with very little else to be done, just cleaning it up and putting a fresh one on, taped down with Microtape.

April 28th

No change. 7.50 a.m. Went for paper but kept all the dressings in place and left it on all day. I could have left it on through the night but changed it just before bedtime. Certainly appears to be working towards a normal colour overall. Anyhow, I have to see the nurse tomorrow so see what she thinks.

April 29th

My appointment is for 10.10 a.m. with the nurse who, after releasing all the tape, which I know I overdo, looked at it and said, 'It will not be necessary for you to make any more appointments with us for it looks fine. Am sure it is now well on the road to making some good healthy tissue.' I said, 'Yes, that's how I feel about it. If only the hole will heal over.' I won't tell you what else I have noted down in the diary for indeed I did have a busy rest of the day. I told her I would like to thank them all at the Health Centre in The Drive for putting up with me over the last few months, and suffering alongside me.

April 30th

After changing my dressing at 7.00 a.m. with nothing untoward occurring, went for paper, did lots of chores. After completing the crossword, I decided to change my dressing at 12.30 hours, as it was beginning to feel uncomfortable. Blood!!! Lots of blood!!! In fact I could not believe so much blood had come out of such a tiny little hole. Anyhow I applied a fair bit of pressure which quickly stopped the flow!!! I have noted, 'Don't know why!!!' Does anyone else, come to think of it? This knocked me for six for the rest of the day. For I had such an important date this coming Thursday for my book launch at the Epping Book Shop at 13.00 hours.

Wednesday, May 1st

I have an appointment with Mr Mac for 15.30 hours. He hardly said a thing after an inspection of the area where the discharge was coming from, telling me, 'Come and see me in a fortnight's time,' and told the nurse to clean it all up and put fresh dressings on. I said I was surprised that he did not want a swab taken. She said, 'He thinks perhaps it does not warrant it.'

May 2nd

My big day—all went according to plan. I made a couple of Victoria sponges for the girls and staff in the bookshop and also for anyone who purchased a book. I did have a very important VIP turn up—the old Essex and England Test Cricketer, Doug Insole with a number of local people I knew, plus friends who had shared some cricket experiences with me!!! Yes, I was mighty pleased that I had made it though none suspected that I was wearing a dressing. The press were there also, taking photos.

May 3rd

I took the dressing off last night and as I had had a few glasses during the evening, never even thinking about my health problems and, this morning, I awoke in bed to feel round my knee for the first time—to find there was nothing on the wound!!! First thought—it must have come off during the night; sitting up in bed I felt all around and under my body. Nothing!!! I turned the sheets back to have a good look at the damage!!!

It was dry!!! I found my spectacles and felt all round the channel where I had experienced discharge for a long time now. It was all dry. I carefully got out of bed, drew the curtains, went to the living room, sat on the settee to find indeed that fate had decided to put me back in the big percentage field, at last.

As you can imagine, through the following days and nights, until my next appointment with Mr Mac on the 15th May, I kept feeling round to make sure that the healing was now progressive. I now started to do some bending and easy quads contractions. Overdoing it I must not do and, after consulting the physio at Holly House Hospital, she said, 'If it's healing all the way down the wound, yes of course do some bending as long as you don't overdo it. Time and patience are the positive words.'

On May 15th I saw Mr Mac at 15.00 hours; he seems highly delighted now that a nightmare for him is over. Over the months I had been involved with him, I didn't expect him to dance around the floor, or jump up and down. He just stroked his chin a few times, saying, 'Have you done any exercises yet?' Then I told him, 'The one I thought might be helping besides the quads contractions was this one,' showing that I was getting down into a crouched position which was giving me nearly a ninety degrees bend, with both legs in unison. He seemed well pleased with this, saying, 'We shall have to have a blood test done to make doubly sure that the infection has finally been cleared.' I am sure you can understand how relieved I was for it seemed that I would never get away from the Holly House Hospital as much as I enjoyed all the company. Even then, coming out of Outpatients a few who knew me passed on their best wishes. A couple asked me (waitresses), 'When are you coming back in, Perc?' I told them, 'I am pretty sure you are not going to see me for some time, now that I have been given the green discharge action light.'

During my long stay at Holly House Hospital, there have been innumerable incidents that have made my life within the four walls so bearable with something different occurring almost every day. Two such jovial occurrences quickly come to mind.

This particular afternoon, I received a visit from Pultzer who had almost mastered the blood pressure equipment, and when there were quiet times would pop in to experiment on my arm. Of course, as we all know, if those bags are not placed correctly around your arm muscles and the squeezing of the bulb starts, be prepared. On one occasion, with one eye on the equipment, the other on getting the pumping action correct, Pultzer had done everything right, except that the air somehow would not work together with the bulk. The air was coming out all over the place, so I put my newspaper down and said, 'What on earth are you up to?' as the pipe had found its way down my side and was roving about under the bedclothes, its emissions concocting all sorts of shapes beneath the bedlinen. The head of nursing walked in. Panic! Not at all. Pultzer walked calmly to the switch on the wall, turned the whole thing off and walked out, closing the door. The director of nursing straightaway said, 'What a polite nurse she is.'

I knew why she had come—to thank me for the letter of condolence I had sent her a few days previously.

When it was all clear again, Pultzer returned, and I told her how the director of nursing had sung her praises, saying what a very polite nurse she was, and awarding her high marks for her courtesy.

I don't mind telling you we have had some laughs about this episode, when the blood pressure equipment decided to go haywire.

In Room 151, quite often when there was a change over, the various nurses made up their charts, or log books as I called them, so quite often the log would not get back to the bottom of the bed where it is usually kept clipped to the bottom rail. It is kept there so that it can be easily removed, looked at, checked by whoever and put back again. Today it had been left outside. On one particular afternoon at approximately 14.30 hours, a new nurse came in, looking for my chart. I said to her, 'If it isn't in the room, it's probably outside lying against the half-closed door in the corridor.' I do know it was about the time when my chart book had also warranted a changeover, for it had got filled up with all the marking up which went on day and night. A new one had replaced it certainly, so presumably the changeover nurses had not noticed this; this caused some alarm for twenty minutes or so. With myself considering this document could be very valuable in years to come, and seeing the RSM go past, just as one of the waitresses together with the new nurse were even looking in my locker, wondering where Percy's chart had gone to, I exclaimed, 'That's who's taken it. She knows it's going to be worth a lot of money, that's who's taken it,' and pointed to the RSM, standing there holding a tray with not a clue as to what was taking place. Until I told her that my chart had been mislaid and, 'You know it's worth a lot of money. You had better own up and tell us what you have done with it.' Of course, RSM cottoned on right away with the now more than a little confused nurse again searching for the chart.

Again my room was carefully searched (pretty sure she had not a clue) with no luck. A staff nurse came in to say, 'Both books have been found, so all is well.' With a big beaming smile appearing on the new nurse's face, she said, 'I did not think she would want to take your chart, Mr Percy.' Of course now it was my turn for the surprise, for she must have understood every word. RSM had long gone, and when she turned up again with a pot of tea and a slice of fruit cake she said, 'You know, Perc, that book of yours might well be worth a lot of money in a few years' time.' I said, 'I've a good mind to make management an offer—to purchase that chart and then flog it to the highest bidder.' Quick as a flash, her reply: 'I should want a cut, Perc.'

Part of a letter I received from Snowy on March 12th, 2002.

The Consultant's Advice

He was telling me about a swelling he had had for several weeks in his left foot—thinking it was another case of gout, he decided to fix an appointment with Mr Drake, a consultant who was a jolly type, which lessened the fear of any visit.

'On arrival he said, "Trouble? Sit down."

' "Yes," was the reply, "it's my foot, all red and painful, and swollen as you can see." Straightaway Mr Drake went to the computer, tapping at the keyboard, all very modern and up to date, I thought.

' "Right!" Mr Drake's voice seemed as if he had resolved the problem: "Get over to the window." The window—a large bay one about ten feet away. I hobbled over painfully to the windowsill as per instructions.

' "Okay, face the pane of glass and put your tongue out, maybe a dozen times, put the fingers of both hands in your ears and move them about, say, in up and down movements." I did as I was asked.

' "Right, come back to the desk and sit down." I painfully hobbled back. Straightaway he was typing away on his computer.

'I said, "It's good to see that the old methods of medicine and such like are equally as important as modern methods."

' "How do you mean?" Mr Drake asked.

' "Well I have come in with my foot problem and straightaway you presumably have gone to your computer with my tongue helping in some way to cure my pains, it certainly seems better."

'Mr Drake looked at me and said, "You poking your tongue out has bugger all to do with your gout. I just don't like the consultant across the road!!" '

Healing At Last

It does not matter what department of Holly House Hospital I have been associated with or which category they fall in, from administration down to the porters, I cannot find enough positive words to describe each and every one: bright, cheerful, willing to listen, understanding, commiserating, full of suggestions, ideas, friendly; the list as far as words go are endless. New nurses on the block quickly get the idea that to make a patient smile or laugh is the way forward. Then it's guaranteed that the response is past all expectations, even for the One-Per-Centers. I am sure you will agree. I am now well on the road to recovery, with only the bending of the leg to work on, which needs a lot of exercise.

The other leg has a movement of something like 115 degrees, now that's a fair bit of difference, compared with the recently repaired one with its 90 degrees movement!! I am constantly being told that I must persevere, for this is the only way it will get back to normal. It's not as though I have been idle, regarding working on it. As soon as I was confident that I could start putting more strain on the repaired knee, first thing in the mornings before I got out of bed, I did quads contractions, followed by a spell on the settee with weights tied round my ankle (plastic water bottles) then finally about ten minutes with some ice cubes placed in a couple of Sainsbury's carrier bags. Then my crouching position with up and down movements. Then towards the end of September, Chris let me borrow her Kettler Pacer Stationary bicycle. I am still unable to get a complete movement of the pedals going over in unison and that is ten months after my discharge.

Have I given up? Not on your nelly!!! I have visited Holly House Hospital physio department, had visits from the NHS physios and various help and advice from several knowledgeable people. As two or three have pointed out, I must be thankful, after those five major operations to be able to bend it as much as I am doing. Which is a credit to all those concerned.

Postscript

As I reach the final part of the script of *One Per Cent*, when the words 'closing down' mean just that an important disclosure has reached my ears and eyes—this week ending October 11th 2003.

It seems a new hip replacement technique called a two-incision operation has been pioneered; this can reduce a patient's stay in hospital quite considerably, and has been developed in America.

Now it has been advanced in the United Kingdom—by three orthopaedic surgeons, who have been specifically trained for this procedure. Our own Mr McAuliffe is one of this trio! Isn't this tremendous news?!!!

And he has said to the local press: 'This is an exciting development in surgery, which offers real advantages to patients—minimally invasive surgery causes less pain, less blood loss, and less muscle damage; patients get better more quickly, and of course go home sooner—reducing the conventional times of about eleven days—to three days.

All of us who have been through his very capable hands wish him every success with his future work and continuing dedication.

Answers to Cricket Questions from Lords' Test Matches

---

1. Typhoon Tyson.
2. England v South Africa 2nd Test, 1955; England won by 71 runs.
3. P B H May, 112 runs.
4. 1958: England v New Zealand, all out, 47 runs..
5. Brian Statham: 1955 England v South Africa 29—12—39—7 wickets.
6. 1926, W Bardsley, 193 not out, match drawn, 2nd Test, England v Australia.
7. This was the one and only time he played for England, 53—24—91—1 wicket.
8. 1964, 17th time, 25—8—48—5 wickets.
9. LEATHER JACKETS.
10. 1968.
11. 5 hrs 20 mins; when he was out to a great catch at Cover by the captain, Percy Chapman. It was said to be the first time that he had lifted the ball in the entire innings. Australia won by 7 wickets.
12. The Year the 6-Ball Over was introduced—1900. A 4-Ball Over had been the norm up until 1889, then it was changed to a 5-Ball one! The 6-Ball Over had been used in Australia since 1887, but it was not for another ten years that 6-Ball Overs came to our shores.

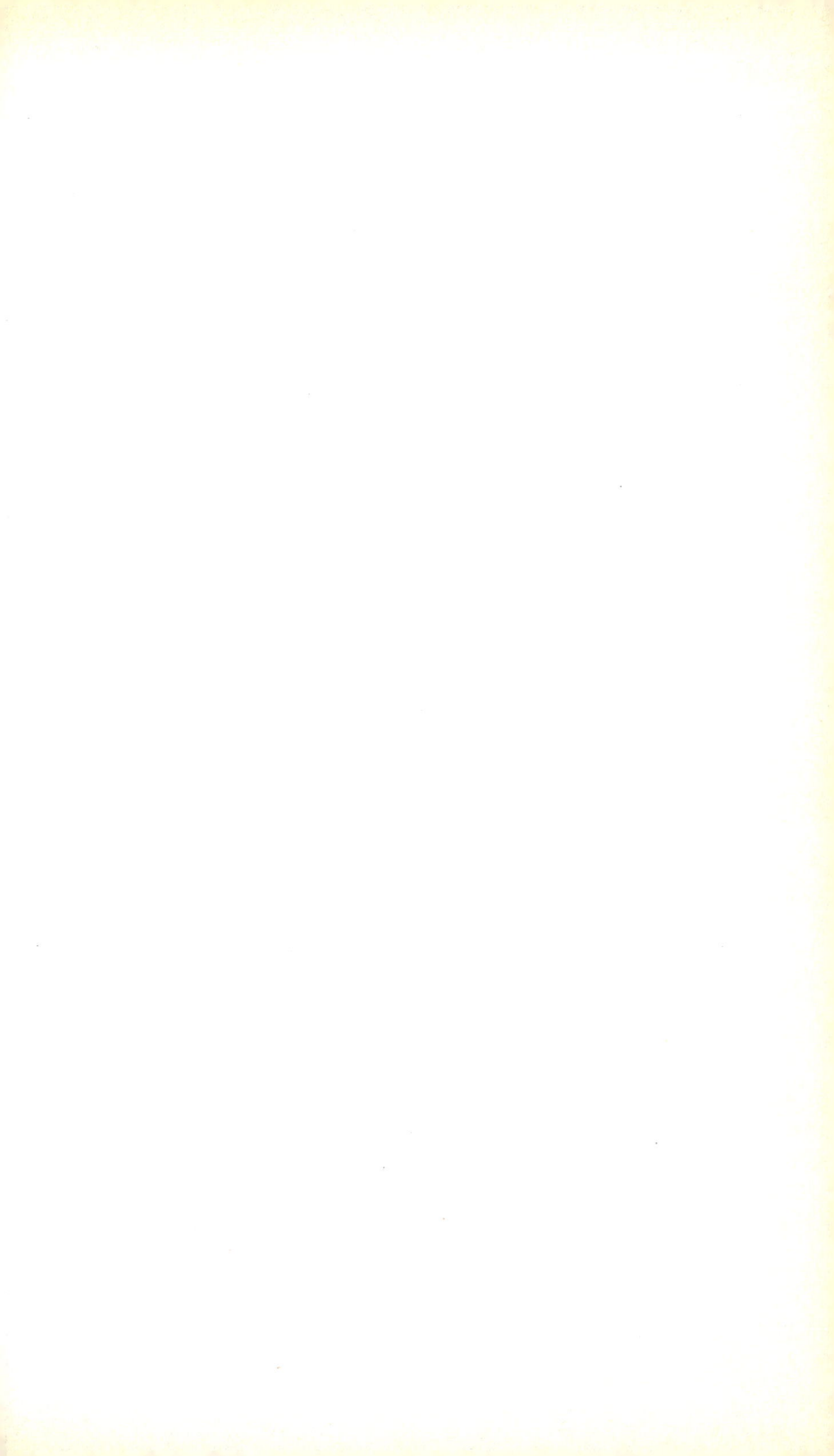